CANCER ETIOLOGY, DIAGNOSIS AND TREATMENTS

HANDBOOK OF SKIN CARE
IN
CANCER PATIENTS

CANCER ETIOLOGY, DIAGNOSIS AND TREATMENTS

Additional books in this series can be found on Nova's website
under the Series tab.

Additional E-books in this series can be found on Nova's website
under the E-books tab.

CANCER ETIOLOGY, DIAGNOSIS AND TREATMENTS

HANDBOOK OF SKIN CARE
IN
CANCER PATIENTS

PIERRE VEREECKEN
AND
AHMAD AWADA
EDITORS

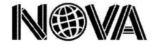

Nova Science Publishers, Inc.
New York

Library of Congress Cataloging-in-Publication Data

Handbook of skin care in cancer patients / editors, Pierre Vereecken, Ahmad Awada.
    p. ; cm.
 Includes bibliographical references and index.
 ISBN 978-1-61668-419-8 (hardcover)
 1. Cancer--Chemotherapy--Complications. 2. Antineoplastic agents--Side effects. 3. Skin--Diseases--Treatment. 4. Skin--Care and hygiene. I. Vereecken, Pierre. II. Awada, Ahmad.
 [DNLM: 1. Neoplasms--complications--Handbooks. 2. Skin Care--Handbooks. 3. Antineoplastic Agents--adverse effects--Handbooks. 4. Neoplasms--drug therapy--Handbooks. 5. Skin Diseases--Handbooks. QZ 39 H2365 2010]
 RC271.C5H37 2010
 616.99'4061--dc22
                             2010013752

Published by Nova Science Publishers, Inc. ✛ *New York*

CONTENTS

Preface   vii

Chapter 1   The Hand-foot Syndrome   1
                Laurent Mortier

Chapter 2   Management of Acneiform Eruption and other Cutaneous
                Side Effects of Anti-EGFR Therapies   9
                Siegfried Segaert and Eric Van Cutsem

Chapter 3   How to Manage Hair Changes in Cancer Patients   21
                *C. Piérard-Franchimont, P. Quatresooz, A. Rorive
                and G. Piérard*

Chapter 4   Nail Changes in Cancer Patients: From Diagnosis to Management   35
                Josette André and Bertrand Richert

Chapter 5   Cancer and Photoprotection   51
                *Christelle Comte,
                and Bernard Guillot*

Chapter 6   A Critical Review of Cutaneous Toxicity of Anticancer Treatments   63
                Hans Prenen and Ahmad Awada

Chapter 7   Pressure Ulcers of Cancer Patients   79
                Patricia Senet and Olivier Chosidow

Chapter 8   How Dermatopathology Can Be Useful in the Comprehension
                of Therapeutic and Side Effects of Novel Biologically
                Targeted Therapies   89
                Laporte Marianne

Chapter 9   The Common and the Unusual Presentation of Skin Metastases
                in Cancer Patients   95
                Wolfram Fink and Dirk Schadendorf

Chapter 10 Cosmetic and Medicinal Products: A Distinct
                but Complementary Approach...?   117
                Alain Lechien

Chapter 11   Management of Lower Limb edema in Cancer Patients   **129**
                  Leduc Olivier, Delathouwer Olivier, Titeca Géraldine,
                  Vereecken Pierre and Leduc Albert

Chapter 12   Keloids and Hypertrophic Scars after Surgery in Cancer Patients **139**
                  D. Franck, A. De Mey and W. D. Boeckx

Chapter 13   Cytotoxic Drug Extravasation in Cancer Patients:
                  Diagnosis, Prevention and Management   **149**
                  Yassine Lalami

Chapter 14   Skin Manifestations of Paraneoplastic Syndromes   **163**
                  Jean Klastersky, Maria-Letizia Cappelletti,
                  Florence Neczyporenko and Marie-Therese Genot

Chapter 15   Tattoos and Camouflage: Not to Forget!   **183**
                  Dachelet Claire and Titeca Géraldine ,
                  Comas Marine, Steels Emmanuelle
                  and Vereecken Pierre

Appendix 1   Common Terminology Criteria for Adverse Events (CTCAE)
                  Version 4.02 (Adapted from U.S. Department of Health
                  and Human Services, National Institutes of Health,
                  National Cancer Institute   **185**

Index   **195**

PREFACE

During the past decade, fundamental and clinical research have been conducted to enhance the efficacy of anticancer treatments and new drugs targeted on specific molecular events have emerged. These treatments are more efficient but also cause frequent skin side effects such as skin dryness, nail and hair changes. On a psychological and aesthetic point of view, this can be a real matter for the patients, and these skin changes lead to altered quality of life and modification of the self perception of the body. This book reviews research conducted on the topic of skin care in cancer patients

Chapter 1 - The hand-foot syndrome (HFS), also known as palmoplantar erythrodysesthesia is a side effect, which can occur with several types of chemotherapy or biologic therapy drugs used to treat cancer. HFS is usually self limiting and rarely leads to hospitalization or life-threatening manifestations. However, if it is not recognized early and managed effectively, an initially mild, cutaneous reaction can progress to an extremely painful condition with a considerable impact on patient's quality of life. For these reasons, early recognition and management of this skin toxicity is crucial in the management of patients. In this chapter, author will describe clinical presentation and physiopathology of HFS. Author will also propose recommendation for prevention and treatment of HFS.

Chapter 2 - EGFR-targeted therapies (monoclonal antibodies such as cetuximab and panitumumab as well as tyrosine kinase inhibitors like erlotinib and gefitinib) are responsible for a unique constellation of mechanism-based, class-specific side effects on the skin. Besides the well known acneiform eruption, this skin toxicity consists of xerosis (leading to eczema and fissures), paronychia, hair changes, telangiectasia, hyperpigmentation and mucosal changes. Dermatologic treatment is supportive and aims at maintaining quality of life while continuining EGFR-inhibitor therapy. Although a recent study demonstrated the effectiveness of prophylactic minocycline in cetuximab-induced acneiform eruption, randomized controlled trials remain sparse and evidence-based guidelines are lacking. Based on personal experience, most cases of acneiform eruption are well controlled by topical metronidazole and oral minocycline 100 mg qd. For severe reactions, mincocycline dose is doubled and saline compresses have proven very valuable. For superinfection with *Staphylococcus aureus* oral cefuroxim axetil can be added for a short term. Emollients and topical steroids can be administered for skin dryness or eczema. Paronychia is the hardest part to treat but antiseptic soaks and a corticosteroid paste can alleviate symptoms to some degree.

Chapter 3 - Cancer patients under treatment develop quite frequently changes in the density and structure of hair fibres. These alterations mainly result from modifications in the germinative compartment of the hair matrix and in the relationship between melanocytes and trichocytes. As a result hair effluvium and alopecia ensue, but also conversally hypertrichosis and trichomegaly. The hair colour and hair shape are not unfrequently altered. There is no radioprotective agent active against ionizing radiations. In case of short term cytostatic perfusion, scalp hypothermia procedures and tourniquet pressure can help reducing the impact on hair growth. Minoxidil has no preventive effect, but it is susceptible to reduce the severity and duration of cytostatic-induced alopecia. Anyway, any psychological support is always important for the patient. Wearing a wig should be encouraged when needed.

Chapter 4 - Nail involvement during chemotherapy is common. Because of the kinetic of nail formation, the nail changes appear several weeks after drug intake. They are characterized by the involvement of several nails, rarely all twenty nails, more often on the fingers than on the toes. Clinical presentation depends on the duration and severity of the toxic injury as well as on the nail component involved, and may result in Beau's lines, onychomadesis, longitudinal melanonychia, onycholysis or pyogenic granuloma. The pathogenesis of nail damage is often not fully understood. These side effects disappear upon cessation of the treatment with the offending drug. They however rarely alter the patient's quality of life and do not impose treatment discontinuance, except occasionally when the most recent chemotherapeutic drugs are involved (taxanes and epidermal growth factor receptor (EGFR) inhibitors). Management is very conservative and mostly orientated towards adequate nail care, in order to help the patient overcome these side effects until the chemotherapy is completed

Chapter 5 - Patients undergoing treatment for a cancer don't know which attitude to adopt with the sun. Indeed, some treatments can be very sensitizing and may cause skin burns, even when the exposure occurs before the start of the cure. This chapter attempts to list these treatments. Too much exposure to the sun can also cause skin cancers and patients need to know how to protect themselves. Paradoxically however, sun may also contribute in fighting against the tumoral proliferative process, via synthesis of vitamin D, which is one of the fundamental hormones for our immune system

Chapter 6 - Cutaneous reactions to chemotherapy are very common in clinical practice and may contribute significantly to the morbidity of cancer patients. Therefore, recognition and management of these side effects is important to provide optimal care. Chemotherapy-related cutaneous toxicity includes generalized rashes as well as site specific toxicity such as mucositis, nail changes or for example hand-foot syndrome. Most of these toxic effects are reversible with delay or dose reductions of chemotherapy. Newer anticancer targeted therapies may also be associated with cutaneous toxicity. In this chapter authors would like to give an overview of the most common cutaneous side effects of classical chemotherapy as well as the new monoclonal antibodies and tyrosine kinase inhibitors.

Chapter 7 - Pressure ulcers are ischemic tissue damages, localised to the skin and the underlying tissues. They are mainly caused by extrinsic factors such as interface pressure, in patients presenting autonomy impairment. Pressure ulcer prevalence varies greatly by clinical setting but remains high, up to 10,5% in hospitals. The Norton Scale and the Braden Scale are the principal prediction tools for evaluating individual patient risk for pressure ulcer development, when used as an adjunct to the clinical judgement. Prevention and treatment are based on skin and local wound care, repositionning, use of pressure relieving support surfaces, nutritional support and surgery in some cases and for selcted localizations as trochanteric area. Pressure ulcers are associated with an increase in mortality rates, and health costs. Thus, prevention is critical to reduce their prevalence in hospital settings and long term care

Chapter 8 - Dermatology and dermatopathology could provide some useful tools in the management of anti-EGFR treatments from two points of view: -clinical symptoms such as rash can be the signal of effectiveness of treatments by cetuximab,ABX-EGF and erlonitib.-immunochemistry on skin samples could give informations on Ki67 and p27 kip1 expression in the skin during treatment, which is probably the reflect of 'what's going on'in the tumor.

Chapter 9 - Cutaneous metastases are an infrequent sign of advanced internal malignancies but may in some cases be the first opportunity to diagnose a so far unapparent cancer. Their early detection may significantly accelerate the initiation of a stage related therapy for a potentially treatable cancer. Moreover may these skin metastases serve as an easily accessible source of tumor cells in the era of adapted and specific tumor therapy. Virtually any body site can be involved, but more common sites of cutaneous metastasis are the scalp, umbilicus, chest wall, and abdominal wall. Uncommon findings are metastases to the nail bed, eye-lid, scars or benign skin lesions. The typical presentation are painless nodules, but mimicry of other cutaneous disorders has hampered diagnosis in many cases. Frequencies of cutaneous metastasis roughly correspond to the overall incidence of the various visceral malignancies, with carcinomas of the lung, breast, colon, and melanoma leading. But basically any tumor can metastasize to the skin and an exhaustive number of case reports has been published on cutaneous metastasis of rare malignancies. Even though they may occur at any time point in the course of the disease, most frequently detection of skin metastases follows the diagnosis of the primary tumor and is an ominous sign of advanced disease. Both, very early and very late metastasis to the skin has been observed, the interval between primary and metastatic diagnosis ranging from less than one week to more than twenty years. Given the therapeutic and prognostic value of an early diagnosis of cutaneous metastases, knowledge about the common and uncommon features is crucial for clinicians in charge of cancer patients.

Chapter 10 - Differentiating a cosmetic product from a medicinal product is not always easy, especially as there are many misconceptions on the subject. This article defines cosmetic and medicinal products within a European context both in relation to each other and in relation to biocidal products and medical devices.The significance of cosmetic products is also examined.

Chapter 11 - Lower limb edema remains the most common complication after cancer treatment that produces an obstruction of the lymphatic system resulting in a decreased draining capacity. The authors describe briefly the physiology and physiopathology of the lymphatic system even as the etiology and the stages of the edema. The physical treatment of the edema is described during and after the hospitalization.Finally, the surgical treatment of the edema is also evoked.

Chapter 12 - After a dermal injury, the biochemical process of wound repair initiates a complex series of events that results in the deposition of a collagen-rich matrix. In certain individuals, the repair process may be pathologic and result in large, raised collagenous scars known as keloids or hypertrophic scars, both characterized by excessive collagen deposition. The two key differences between keloid and hypertrophic scar are the 'time-line' and the association with contraction. The pathogenesis of keloids is complex and involves both genetic and environmental factors. Although there is no single definitive treatment modality, there are numerous therapeutic regiments that have been described. In the authors' own experience the application of 24 hours per day pressure therapy, especially for hypertrophic facial burns scars , during an eighteen months period, has proven to be effective and authors have published the good results of brachytherapy for the treatment of keloids of variable origin. A broad revue of the literature about keloids shows that there is no publication demonstrating an increased risk to develop keloids after cancer surgery but well an increased risk of infection and wound healing delay because of the immune and nutritional status of the patient and those are two important risk factors for the development of keloid scars.

Chapter 13 - Chemotherapy remains a cornerstone for the treatment of cancer, either for solid and haematological malignancies, in early and advanced stage disease. The very great majority of cytotoxic drugs are administered by intravenous perfusions. Moreover, various toxicities are associated to anticancer chemotherapy, depending on the type of cytotoxic agent considered. Such acute or delayed toxicities are currently well managed, allowing a preservation of patient's quality of life during the scheduled treatment. However, cytotoxic drug extravasation can be considered as an iatrogenic complication well described in the literature, but also probably underestimated and understudied, with a clear lack of general consensus for the medical management, even if practical rules are being developed in clinical institutions.

Chapter 14 - Acrokeratosis paraneoplastica, hypertrichosis lanuginosa, erythema gyratum repens, hypertrophic osteoarhtropathy, dermatomyositis and Sweet's syndrome are often – although not always- associated with a malignant tumor. Recognition of any of these potential paraneoplastic skin disorders should lead to a strong suspicion for an occult malignancy and trigger appropriate work-up. In case of negative investigation, a high suspicion level for an occult malignancy must be maintained for years. Paraneoplastic skin manifestations with well known pathophysiological mechanisms related to a tumor, such as cutaneous amyloidosis, melanic pigmentation, vasculitis, carcinoid flushing, hirsutism, gynecomastia and others, can be responsible for signs and symptoms requiring specific therapies. These manifestations ususaly follow a course that is clearly related to that of the tumor and can thus serve as surrogates for its evolution.

Chapter 15 - Cosmetic skin care including tattoos and camouflages is an important issue in cancer patients, and these techniques have to be considered as a powerful help in many patients. The medical tattoo allows the aesthetic repair of some areas of the body and quite specifically lips and breast, and eyelids. This is obtained thanks to the use of pigments of iron oxide with a wide choice of colors.

In: Handbook of Skin Care in Cancer Patients
Editors: Pierre Vereecken and Ahmad Awada

ISBN: 978-1-61668-419-8
© 2012 Nova Science Publishers, Inc.

Chapter 1

THE HAND-FOOT SYNDROME

*Laurent Mortier**

Clinique de Dermatologie, Hôpital Huriez, CHRU Lille, Rue Michel Polonovski,
59037 Lille Cedex, France

ABSTRACT

The hand-foot syndrome (HFS), also known as palmoplantar erythrodysesthesia is a side effect, which can occur with several types of chemotherapy or biologic therapy drugs used to treat cancer.

HFS is usually self limiting and rarely leads to hospitalization or life-threatening manifestations. However, if it is not recognized early and managed effectively, an initially mild, cutaneous reaction can progress to an extremely painful condition with a considerable impact on patient's quality of life.

For these reasons, early recognition and management of this skin toxicity is crucial in the management of patients.

In this chapter, we will describe clinical presentation and physiopathology of HFS. We will also propose recommendation for prevention and treatment of HFS.

INTRODUCTION

The hand-foot syndrome (HFS), also known as palmoplantar erythrodysesthesia is a side effect, which can occur with several types of chemotherapy or biologic therapy drugs used to treat cancer. Elicitation of an HFS by antineoplastic chemotherapy was first described by Zuehlke in 1974 with mitotane therapy [1].

Practically every chemotherapeutic agent has been found to be associated with HFS (in either isolated cases or small series of patients), and it is sometimes difficult to assess the true effect of a particular agent because combination therapies are now widely used. The most commonly implicated chemotherapeutic agents are 5-fluorouracil, doxorubicin, cytarabine,

---

* Correspondence: Tel : + 33.3.20.44.41.93; Fax : + 33.3.20.44.59.16; Email : l-mortier@chru-lille.fr

docetaxel. More recently HFS has also been described with target therapy such as sorafenib and imatinib [2,3].

The actual incidence of HFS is very difficult to determine because most reports in literature are isolated or short case series. Moreover, in large series cutaneous reaction are usually mentioned with few details. However, HFS can affect up to 34% of patients receiving continuous 5-fluorouracil infusion and 13% of those receiving bolus 5-fluorouracil [4-6]. The rate of occurrence of HFS is similar for continuous 5-fluorouracil infusion and capecitabine, an oral prodrug of 5-fluorouracil [7]. Capecitabine, however, is now one of the leading causes of HFS as it is more widely used than 5-fluorouracil.

There is no evidence in the literature that HFS prefers a race or population group. It can occur in children and adults, and there are no known gender differences.

HFS is usually self limiting and rarely leads to hospitalization or life-threatening manifestations. However, if it is not recognized early and managed effectively, an initially mild, cutaneous reaction can progress to an extremely painful condition with a considerable impact on patient's quality of life. Moreover HFS is the most common chemotherapy-induced dose-limiting toxic skin reaction. Indeed, it is the most serious dose limiting effect of treatments involving oral capecitabine (Figure 1, 2).

For these reasons, early recognition and management of this skin toxicity is crucial in the management of patients.

CLINICAL PRESENTATION

HFS follows a practically identical clinical course in all patients, whatever the causative agent. It is characterized by the appearance of erythema, swelling, which may be accompanied in severe cases with edema, blistering, erosions or, infrequently, ulcerations (Figure 1, 2). The lateral sides of fingers or the periungual zones can also be affected.

Table 1. Clinical Classification of HFS

NCI-CTC Scale		WHO Scale	
Grade	Definition	Grade	Definition
1	Skin changes without pain (erythema, peeling)	1	Dysesthesias/paresthesias, tingling in palms and soles
2	Skin changes with pain, not interfering with function	2	Discomfort holding objects and upon walking; erythema or painless swelling of palms and soles
3	Skin changes with pain, interfering with function	3	Painful edema and erythema; periungual erythema and swelling
		4	Peeling, blisters, ulcerations; severe pain

CTC: common toxicity criteria.
NCI: National Cancer Institute.
WHO: World Health Organization.

Symptoms typically start 48 hours after chemotherapy administration and most patients experience localized discomfort intolerance to contact with hot objects before the skin lesions appear. Soles tend to be less severely affected than palms, and lesions are often more evident on the fleshy parts and pressure areas. Lesions last for 1 to 2 weeks and get increasingly worse with additional cycles. After withdrawal of the chemotherapy, symptoms disappeared in few days and healing is observed in a few days without scars, as long as there was no ulceration.

Superinfections with Staphylococci or gram-negative bacteria or the occurrence of erysipelas have been observed as complications.

HFS may appear in atypical areas such as the dorsum of the hands and feet, heels and elbows, and even the ears and genital areas [8].

HFS severity can be rated using different classification systems. The 2 most common systems used in clinical practice are the WHO and NCI scales. While the WHO system measures clinical severity, the NCI system measures the level of discomfort experienced by patients. Level of discomfort generally correlates with the clinical appearance of lesions, suggesting that there is a good level of agreement between both grading systems (Table 1).

A PARTICULAR CLINICAL PRESENTATION: HFS INDUCED BY SORAFENIB

Elucidation of dysregulated signaling pathways implicated in tumor development has changed our approach to cancer treatment, resulting in the development of anti-cancer 'targeted agents'. Several targeted agents have been approved for advanced cancer and are revolutionizing the management of patients with solid tumors with previously poor prognosis and limited treatment options. Preclinical studies have shown that sorafenib acts on the tumor (inhibition of proliferation; induction of apoptosis) and tumor vasculature (inhibition of angiogenesis) [3].

Sorafenib has been approved for clear cell renal carcinoma and for hepatocarcinoma and is currently evaluated in phase II/III trials in other cancers.

In a Phase II trial, 93% of patients with renal cell carcinoma receiving sorafenib (400 mg bid) had dermatologic symptoms, including HFS in 62% of cases.

Although sorafenib-induced HFS may sometimes be indistinguishable from classical hand–foot syndrome, it is typically associated with hyperkeratosis in 54% of patients with HFS [3] (Figure 3). The hyperkeratosis presented as painful, patchy keratodermia restricted to pressure areas, whereas classical HFS lesions are often diffuse and less restricted to pressure areas.

PHYSIOPATHOLOGY AND HISTOLOGY

The precise mechanisms which lead to the onset of HFS are largely unknown to date. However, the most likely and widely accepted hypothesis is that chemotherapeutic agents have a direct adverse effect on epidermal cells and particularly basal keratinocytes [9]. This hypothesis rests on the relationship between dose and lesion severity [10] and histopathologic similarities with other conditions caused by direct epidermal cytotoxicity [9].

Why these pathological changes appear primarily on the palms of the hands and soles of the feet has not yet been clarified. Possibly, it is related to specific factors in this preferential localization as: an elevated keratinocyte turn-over rate, a specific microvascularization anatomy, an abundance of eccrine glands, or a temperature gradient [9].

While no large studies have systematically reported histopathologic findings for HFS, there are many reports of isolated cases reported histopathologic changes. More often, these descriptions reveals degeneration of the basement membrane, necrosis in isolated basal keratinocytes, and relative atrophy of the stratum spinosum. Occasional findings include abnormal maturation of keratinocytes, atypical mitosis, multinucleated cells and nuclear aberrations. Other remarkable findings include vascular dilation in the dermis and eccrine gland alterations in the form of eccrine squamous syringometaplasia [11,12].

TREATMENT

In treatment schedules with an expected rate of HFS, it is important that patients are able to use preventive treatment and to recognize early symptoms in order to start therapy or treatment modification without delay.

Prevention

Prevention is very important in trying to reduce the development of hand-foot syndrome. Indeed, patient education is key in the early detection of HFS to minimize discomfort and complications.

Actions taken to prevent hand-foot syndrome will help to reduce the severity of symptoms. This involves modifying some activities to reduce friction and heat exposure (Table 2).

Table 2. Recommendations to patients for prevention of HFS

- Avoid activity increasing pressure on the soles of the feet such as jogging, tennis or long days of walking.
- Avoid prolonged exposure of hands and feet to sources of heat (bathing, washing dishes, sauna…).
- Take cool showers or baths.
- Cool your hands and feet with cool compresses.
- Apply skin care creams to keep your hands moist.
- Wear loose shoes.

Treatment of HFS

Dose reduction, lengthening of administration intervals, and drug withdrawal are the only measures that have proven successful on a regular basis for treatment of HFS. After the first episode of HFS, once the symptoms have abated, therapy can usually be restarted according to the original scheme. If HFS recurs, dose adjustment is mandatory.

Several other methods have been proposed by authors reporting isolated cases and small series, but their efficacy needs to be evaluated in prospective, randomized, controlled studies. Powerful topical corticosteroids have been used with varying levels of success, and the best results have been seen when used in conjunction with cold compresses and emollients [13,14]. Systemic corticosteroids have been successfully used to treat and prevent HFS induced by 5-fluorouracil,liposomal doxorubicin, bleomycin, and methotrexate.

Pyridoxine (vitamin B6) appears to be the most successful treatment [15]. It has also been shown in a canine model that this treatment delayed the onset of HFS and reduced its severity during chemotherapy with liposomal doxorubicin. How this vitamin actually works is unknown but it has been suggested that it might regenerate injured nerve fibers [16].

Cyclooxygenase (COX)-2 inhibition has also been shown effective as a systemic approach for prophylaxis of chemotherapy associated HFS. This response was demonstrated by Lin et al when capecitabine was administered with celecoxib, a cyclooxygenase-2 inhibitor resulted in a decreased incidence of HFS (grade 1: 12.5% versus 34.3%, p = 0.037; grade 2: 3.1% versus 17%) [17]. In this study, a significant increase in the number of patients with stable disease was reported in the group with celecoxib (62.5% versus 22.8%, p = 0.001) [17].

Topical dimethyl sulfoxide, applied 4 times a day over a period of 14 days has been proposed as a treatment for HFS but without sufficient effect [18].

Finally, vitamin E treatment in a small group of patients with HFS improved symptoms [19].

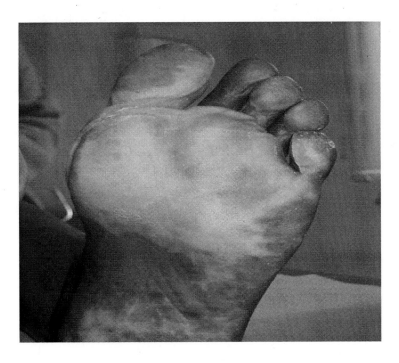

Figure 1. Grade 3 HFS (NCI-CTC scale) induced by capecitabin.

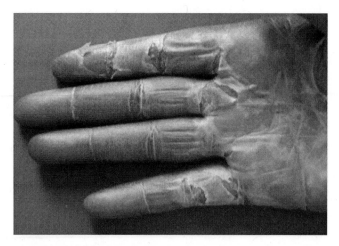

Figure 2. Grade 3 HFS (NCI-CTC scale) induced by capecitabine.

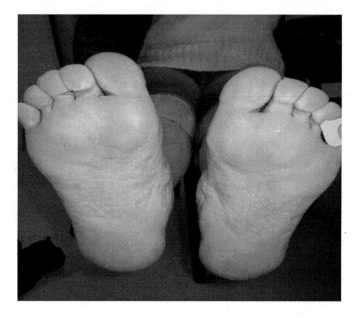

Figure 3. Grade 2 HFS (NCI-CTC scale) induced by sorafenib.

REFERENCES

[1]   Zuehlke RK. Erythematous eruption of the palms and soles associated with mitotane therapy. *Dermatologica.* 1974;148: 90-2.

[2]   Battistella M, Frémont G, Vignon-Pennamen MD, Gornet JM, Dubertret L, Viguier M. Imatinib-induced hand-foot syndrome in a patient with metastatic gastrointestinal-stromal tumor *Arch Dermatol.* 2008 Oct;144(10):1400-2.

[3]   Autier J, Escudier B, Wechsler J, Spatz A, Robert C. Prospective study of the cutaneous adverse effects of sorafenib, a novel multikinase inhibitor. *Arch Dermatol.* 2008 Jul;144(7):886-92.

[4]   Meta-Analysis Group in Cancer. Toxicity of fluorouracil in patients with advanced colorectal cancer: effect of administration schedule and prognostic factors. *J Clin Oncol.* 1998;16: 3537-41.

[5]   Popescu RA, Norman A, Ross PJ, Parikh B, Cunningham D. Adjuvant or palliative chemotherapy for colorectal cancer in patients 70 years or older. *J Clin Oncol.* 1999;17:2412-8.

[6]   Comandone A, Bretti S, LaGrotta G, Manzoni S, Bonardi G, Berardo R, et al. Palmar-plantar erythrodysesthesia syndrome associated with 5-fluorouracil treatment. *Anticancer Res.* 1993;13:1781-3.

[7]   Blum JL, Jones SE, Buzdar AU, LoRusso PM, Kuter I, Vogel C et al. Multicenter phase II study of capecitabine in paclitaxel refractory metastatic breast cancer. *J Clin Oncol.* 1999;17:485-93.

[8]   Sorscher SM. Penile involvement with hand-foot syndrome. *Am J Clin Dermatol.* 2004;5:209-10.

[9]   Fitzpatrick JE. New histopathologic findings in drug eruptions. *Dermatol Clin.* 1992;10:19-36.

[10]   Amantea M, Newman MS, Sullivan TM, Forrest A, Working PK. Relationship of dose intensity to the induction of palmarplantar erythrodysesthesia by pegylated liposomal doxorubicin in dogs. *Hum Exp Toxicol.* 1999;18:17-26.

[11]   Valks R, Fraga J, Porras-Luque J, Figuera A, García-Díaz A, Fernández-Herrera J. Chemotherapy-induced eccrine squamous syringometaplasia. A distinctive eruption in patients receiving hematopoietic progenitor cells. *Arch Dermatol.* 1997;133:873-8.

[12]   Tsuruta D, Mochida K, Hamada T, Ishii M, Wakasa K, Hashimoto S, et al. Chemotherapy induced acral erythema: report of a case and immunohistochemical findings. *Clin Exp Dermatol.* 2000;25:386-8.

[13]   Esteve E, Schillio Y, Vaillant L, Bensaid P, Missonnier F, Metman EH. Efficacité de la corticothérapie séquentielle dans un cas d'érythème acral douloureux secondaire au 5-fluorouracile à fortes doses. *Ann Med Interne (Paris).* 1995;146:192-3.

[14]   Brown J, Burck K, Black D, Collins C. Treatment of cytarabine acral erythema with corticosteroids. *J Am Acad Dermatol.* 1991;24:1023-5.

[15]   Vukelja SJ, Lombardo FA, James WD, Weiss RB. Pyridoxine for the palmar-plantar erythrodysesthesia syndrome. *Ann Intern Med.* 1989;111:688-9.

[16]   Becker KW, Kienecker EW, Dick P. A contribution to the scientific assessment of degenerative and regenerative processes of peripheral nerve fibers following axonotmesis under the systemic administration of vitamins B1, B6 and B12—light and electron microscopy findings of the saphenous nerve in the rabbit. *Neurochirurgia (Stuttg).* 1990;33:113-21.

[17]   Lin E, Morris JS, Ayers GD. Effect of celecoxib on capecitabine induced hand-foot syndrome and antitumor activity. *Oncology (Huntingt)* 2002; 16: 31-7.

[18]   López AM, Wallace L, Dorr RT, Koff M, Hersh EM, Alberts DS. Topical DMSO treatment for pegylated liposomal doxorubicin-induced palmar-plantar erythrodysesthesia. *Cancer Chemother Pharmacol.* 1999;44:303-6.

[19]   Kara IO, Sahin B, Erkisi M. Palmar-plantar erythrodysesthesia due to docetaxel-capecitabine therapy is treated with vitamin E without dose reduction. *Breast.* 2006;15:414-24.

In: Handbook of Skin Care in Cancer Patients
Editors: Pierre Vereecken and Ahmad Awada

ISBN: 978-1-61668-419-8
© 2012 Nova Science Publishers, Inc.

Chapter 2

MANAGEMENT OF ACNEIFORM ERUPTION AND OTHER CUTANEOUS SIDE EFFECTS OF ANTI-EGFR THERAPIES

Siegfried Segaert[1,], and Eric Van Cutsem[2,†]*
[1]Department of Dermatology, University Hospital Leuven, Belgium
[2]Digestive Oncology Unit, University Hospital Leuven, Belgium

ABSTRACT

EGFR-targeted therapies (monoclonal antibodies such as cetuximab and panitumumab as well as tyrosine kinase inhibitors like erlotinib and gefitinib) are responsible for a unique constellation of mechanism-based, class-specific side effects on the skin. Besides the well known acneiform eruption, this skin toxicity consists of xerosis (leading to eczema and fissures), paronychia, hair changes, telangiectasia, hyperpigmentation and mucosal changes. Dermatologic treatment is supportive and aims at maintaining quality of life while continuining EGFR-inhibitor therapy. Although a recent study demonstrated the effectiveness of prophylactic minocycline in cetuximab-induced acneiform eruption, randomized controlled trials remain sparse and evidence-based guidelines are lacking. Based on personal experience, most cases of acneiform eruption are well controlled by topical metronidazole and oral minocycline 100 mg qd. For severe reactions, mincocycline dose is doubled and saline compresses have proven very valuable. For superinfection with *Staphylococcus aureus* oral cefuroxim axetil can be added for a short term. Emollients and topical steroids can be administered for skin dryness or eczema. Paronychia is the hardest part to treat but antiseptic soaks and a corticosteroid paste can alleviate symptoms to some degree.

---

[*] Siegfried.Segaert@med.kuleuven.be
[†] eric.vancutsem@uz.kuleuven.ac.be

CUTANEOUS SIDE EFFECTS OF ANTI-EGFR THERAPIES

The last few years, epidermal growth factor receptor (EGFR) inhibitors have successfully joint the armamentarium of anti-cancer drugs with an increasing number of indications such as colorectal cancer, head and neck cancer, non-small cell lung cancer and breast cancer.[1] EGFR-targeted drugs consist of monoclonal antibodies to EGFR (cetuximab, panitumumab, matuzumab,…), small-molecule tyrosine kinase inhibitors specific for EGFR (erlotinib, gefitinib), dual kinase inhibitors inhibiting EGFR and HER2 (lapatinib), pan-erbB inhibitors inhibiting EGFR and other erbB receptors (canertinib) and others such as vandetanib inhibiting EGFR, VEGFR and RET.[1]

Probably due to the abundant expression of EGFR in the epidermis and its appendages (hair follicles, sebaceous glands), all these EGFR-inhibitors are responsible for a number of class-specific side effects on the skin occurring in most of the patients.[2,3,4] The clinical pattern of EGFR-inhibitor skin toxicity is entirely unique and consists of an acneiform eruption (a sterile, sometimes itchy, follicular papulopustular rash confined to the seborrheic areas occurring in 80% of patients), skin dryness leading to eczema and fissures, paronychia, hair changes (esp. trichomegaly of the eyelashes), hyperpigmentation and telangiectasia.[3] In addition, the oral, ocular, nasal and genital mucosa may be involved as well.[2,5] Microscopic evaluation of acneiform lesions shows an early infiltration of the hair follicle with T-lymphocytes, followed by a hyperkeratotic, ectatic appearance of the follicular infundibula and a florid, neutrophilic folliculitis and perifolliculitis.[3]

Dermatologic toxicities of EGFR-inhibitors appear mechanism-based (i.e. linked to inhibition of EGFR in the skin) as they are common for all EGFR-targeted drugs (antibodies, specific and non-specific tyrosine kinase inhibitors), dose dependent and similar to the changes seen in transgenic mice targeting cutaneous EGFR.[3,4] Moreover the intensity of the acneiform eruption may be correlated with the clinical effectiveness of the EGFR-inhibitor indicating that skin toxicity might serve as a pharmacodynamic marker.[6,7] The sequence of events following inactivation of skin EGFR and leading to skin rash remains elusive however.[4]

Acneiform eruption can be classified according to NCI-CTC version 3.0 into grade 1 (mild asymptomatic), grade 2 (moderate symptomatic) and grade 3 (severe disabling rash). Although not evidence-based, often considered too arbitrary and therefore subject to future improvement, this classification may act as a tool to predict EGFR-inhibitor anti-tumor efficacy[6,7] and to guide dermatologic treatment (see below).[8]

DERMATOLOGIC CARE FOR
EGFR-INHIBITOR SKIN TOXICITY

There is a clear medical need for supportive dermatologic treatment of EGFR-inhibitor skin toxicity. The eruption usually affects the visible skin of the face and may cause itch or pain. Therefore, it often causes such a dramatic impact on self-esteem and quality of life that the patient may wish to stop the EGFR-targeted treatment.[3,9,10] But since the drug can be life-extending or maybe life-saving, its cessation is definitely not the first option to consider. This situation contrasts with the classical drug eruption where dermatological advice focuses on identifying and stopping the responsible drug. In patients treated with EGFR-inhibitors, dermatologic care is not causal but supportive and aims at maintaining quality of life while continuing the EGFR-inhibitor.[11]

The oncology nurse plays a central role in patient education and communication about the skin problems that can be encountered during therapy with EGFR-inhibitors.[10] The nurse explains frequently occurring skin problems, the general measures, the do's and the don'ts, the need to immediately contact in case of trouble. Patient brochures and packages with useful samples (sun blocking cream, shower oil, emollient, hand cream) can help with this task.[11]

Mild to moderate cases of acneiform eruption can well be managed by the oncologist/internist with standard treatment regimens (e.g. topical metronidazole ± oral tetracycline). Grade 3 acneiform eruption and other skin manifestations however, require more specialized care by a dermatologist.[3] Indeed, all principles of topical therapy (e.g. appropriate vehicle choice according to acuity of inflammation and skin site) converge in the care for EGFR-inhibitor skin reactions (see below). Hence, a good collaboration between the oncologist/internist and dermatologist is indispensable. The dermatologist should be available for immediate consultation in case of flare up and frequent dermatologic follow up is mostly needed.[3]

GENERAL MEASURES AND TREATMENT PRINCIPLES

As evidence-based controlled trials are still very sparse[12,13], treatment of EGFR-inhibitor skin toxicity mainly relies on reported personal experience[3,14-19], anecdotal or small series case reports[2] and recommendations from expert consensus conferences.[9,20,21] As a result, there are important geographical variations and even inconsistencies in the clinical management of EGFR-inhibitor skin toxicity: e.g. with respect to acneiform eruption, topical corticosteroids are avoided in Europe[11] but are very frequently used in the United States.[20,21]

Adequate sun protective measures (hat, clothes, sun blocking creams) are advised as sun exposure aggravates acneiform eruption[22] and induces hyperpigmentation.[3] The patient is also instructed to avoid skin care products that dry out the skin (like bath foam, shower gel, soap, very hot water) and to switch to bath/shower oil and lukewarm water. An emollient/hand cream can be used on the limbs and hands to prevent xerosis and fissures, especially after bath/shower, swimming or sauna. The use of greasy ointments on the face and trunk is avoided as this may aggravate acneiform eruption.[3] There is anecdotal American experience with the application of cold compresses during EGFR-inhibitor infusion ('cryotherapy') to prevent acneiform eruption.[10]

The right vehicle choice is essential to successful topical treatment of EGFR-inhibitor skin reactions. For an acute pustular or oedematous reaction, drying vehicles like compresses, gels or oil in water creams can be used but emollient ointments are inappropriate as they occlude the skin pores and thus worsen follicular inflammation. In the chronic stage of the eruption with dry, flaky skin, drying vehicles need to be switched to a rich water in oil cream or an ointment to prevent xerosis.[3] Therefore, topical treatment is tailored to the situation of the individual patient and may change during time, meaning that there is no topical treatment scheme that is universally applicable for all patients at all times.[3]

When an EGFR-inhibitor (e.g. cetuximab) is combined with radiotherapy (e.g. for head and neck cancer), the management remains unaltered as the abovementioned therapies are not interfering with radiotherapy.[23]

Recently, increasing attention has been paid to pre-emptive or prophylactic treatment of acneiform eruption, as it occurs in 80% of patients on EGFR-inhibitors. A recent study demonstrated that preventive use of oral tetracycline 500 mg bid left incidence of acneiform eruption almost unchanged but moved it towards the lower severity range.[12] However, as only around 10% of patients develop severe reactions (benefitting most from pre-emptive treatment) and most of the patients respond reasonably well to reactive treatment, there is no reason to adopt such strategy. Moreover, prophylactic treatment might result in loss of skin toxicity as an efficacy marker.[6,7]

TREATMENT OF ACNEIFORM ERUPTION

For the authors, topical metronidazole and oral minocycline are the standard of treatment. As topical therapy, we prefer metronidazole (as a 2% preparation in cetomacrogol cream or as 0,75% Rozex® cream) because of its mildness as it is normally used for the very sensitive skin of rosacea patients.[24] Topical anti-acne agents such as erythromycin, clindamycin and benzoylperoxide are effective[9,16] but much more aggressive as they are meant for young resilient acne skin.[24] Moreover, EGFR-inhibitor-induced acneiform eruption of the face probably shares more characteristics with inflammatory rosacea than with acne. Topical metronidazole can be used twice a day or in between as needed on the first appearance of papulopustular lesions. Topical retinoids (adapalene, tazarotene) are used by some[9] but lack rational (no comedones)[3]. Moreover, tazarotene was recently shown to be ineffective and too irritating for the facial skin in a left-right comparison study.[13] Topical corticosteroids should be avoided in the face and on the trunk as the possible risks in those areas (induction of steroid rosacea or acne, atrophy, telangiectasia, chronic abuse with tachyphylaxis and steroid dependence) outweigh the advantages.[3,9,18] For papulopustular lesions on the scalp, an exception can be made as this skin site – in contrast to the face, chest and upper back - is quite resistant to local steroid side effects. Calcineurin antagonists (tacrolimus or pimecrolimus), being used as first line therapy in some American centres,[15] are effective but their use is hampered by skin irritation and high price (off-label and not reimbursed). Topical menadione (vitamin K3, an EGFR phosphatase inhibitor with promising preclinical properties)[25] is not available yet for clinical use and unsure to meet the expectations. We also instruct the patient to stick to the prescribed topical treatment and discourage the use of all kinds of over the counter products that are marketed for skin irritation (e.g. tea tree oil)[10] but very often cause contact allergy. Camouflage techniques have been used with success to hide the skin changes provoked by EGFR-inhibitors.[14] However, they are not advized in the acute phase of the rash (occlusive effect).

Acneiform eruption-associated itch can easily be controlled with an oral antihistamine of choice (cetirizine, loratadine, hydroxyzine).[3] The initiation of oral tetracyclines is mostly based on clinical judgement (insufficient response to topical metronidazole, extensive disease). The preferred type of tetracycline may vary. Minocycline 100 mg qd is our cycline of choice but it is avoided by some because of the rare occurrence of drug-induced lupus, hepatitis or hyperpigmentation.[9] Doxycycline 100 mg qd (may cause photosensitivity) or lymecycline 300 mg qd are alternatives.[9] Like metronidazole, tetracyclines are not administered for their antibiotic but for their anti-inflammatory properties;[24] usually they are given for months.[3] In case of severe grade 3 reactions, tetracycline dose is doubled until a grade 2 is reached again.[3] For grade 3 reactions with numerous or confluent pustules, extensive exsudation or marked oedema, saline compresses (15 minutes for 2 to 3 times a day) are very helpful for rapid clearance of the inflammation.[3] Compresses dry out the skin very much. Therefore, they should only be applied for a limited duration of time (a few days) and each application should be followed by repeated application of metronidazole cream.

Acneiform eruption by EGFR-inhibitors is essentially sterile but the skin is highly prone to superinfection with *Staphylococcus aureus*.[3] As tetracyclines are rarely active against *S. aureus*, a penicillinase-resistant penicillin (e.g. flucloxacillin 500 mg tid) or cephalosporin (e.g. cefuroxim axetil 500 mg bid) can be added for 5 days; usually a swab is taken, so that the antibiotic can be switched accordingly in case of resistance. Superinfection with *herpes simplex* is rare but requires oral (e.g. aciclovir, valaciclovir) or intravenous (aciclovir) antiviral drugs.[3]

In case of a grade 3 reaction, dermatologic treatment is given while continuing the EGFR-inhibitor at unchanged dose; a re-evaluation then takes place after one week. Very often, a grade 3 acneiform eruption improves so rapidly on dermatologic therapy that there is no need for dose adjustment or interruption of the EGFR-inhibitor. Only in the rare cases (<5% of cases) where a grade 3 reaction is more persisting despite appropriate dermatologic support, the EGFR-inhibitor can be given at a lower dose or can be interrupted until a decrease of skin toxicity grading (personal experience).

Despite its efficacy for EGFR-inhibitor-dependent rash,[17] we plead against the use of oral isotretinoin as it may possibly interfere with EGFR-inhibitor anti-tumor activity by downregulating EGFR expression.[3] Moreover, isotretinoin shares a large number of side effects with EGFR-inhibitors (xerosis, sensitivity for *S. aureus* superinfection, paronychia, pyogenic granuloma), which may lower tolerability.[3] Systemic steroids are also to be avoided to treat acneiform eruption as they may induce a similar eruption themselves; in addition they may hamper the antibody-dependent cell-mediated cytotoxicity that is ascribed to the EGFR-antibody cetuximab.[9]

TREATMENT OF XEROSIS, ECZEMA AND FISSURES

Skin xerosis obviously benefits from the general hydrating measures described above. In addition, an appropriate vehicle choice is indispensable. In this respect, alcoholic lotions or gels for treating acneiform eruption should be discouraged in favour of oil in water creams (e.g. metronidazole cream) and saline compresses for severe rash should be limited in time. On the limbs greasy (water in oil) creams or even ointments can be used for moderate to severe xerosis. The right balance should, however, always be kept since occlusive ointments may facilitate the development of folliculitis lesions.[3]

When eczema is present, a topical weak to medium strength corticosteroid cream is recommended for a short term (one to two weeks). Salicylic acid can be added to the steroid when fingertop eczema is present. When the eczema becomes wet, superinfection should be suspected and a swab for bacterial (or viral) culture can be taken. A treatment with topical (fusidic acid) or in severe cases systemic anti-*S. aureus* antibiotics can be added for 5-10 days (e.g. flucloxacillin 500 mg tid or cefuroxim axetil 500 mg bid). In the rare case of *herpes simplex* superinfection, treatment with systemic antiviral drugs is necessary.[3]

Fissures can be treated with propyleneglycol 50% aqueous solution under plastic occlusion (daily for 30 minutes), salicylic acid 10% ointment, a hydrocolloid dressing or liquid cyanoacrylate glue.[3]

TREATMENT OF PARONYCHIA

Paronychia is often very distressing and painful for the patients as it impedes walking or normal use of the fingers. Unfortunately, paronychia is also very challenging to manage as no treatment yields complete relief. Wearing shoes that are not too tight is an important preventive measure to minimize friction and pressure on the nail fold. Paronychia caused by EGFR-blockers is not infective in nature but renders the nail folds very sensitive to infection. Therefore antiseptic (chloramine, polyvidon iodine) soaks or creams are advized on a daily basis. When superinfection is suspected, swabs can be taken and oral anti-*S. aureus* antibiotics (e.g. flucloxacillin) given. Using an ultrapotent topical steroid cream on the nail folds at the earliest signs of paronychia may prevent it from worsening. On settled paronychia, a drying paste containing an antiseptic (chlorhexidine), an anti-yeast (nystatin) and a potent topical corticosteroid can be helpful in alleviating symptoms.[3] Oral tetracyclines can be helpful as well in treating paronychia.[26] Oral non steroidal anti-inflammatory drugs can be administered to control the pain. Silver nitrate application on a weekly basis improves pyogenic granuloma. Despite the clinical appearance mimicking an ingrown nail, partial nail bed excision has no effect on EGFR-inhibitor-caused paronychia. Total nail extraction with destruction of nail matrix cures the paronychia but the permanent loss of the nail limits the usefulness of this technique. In severe, recalcitrant cases, interruption of the EGFR-blocker may be considered; but just like it takes many weeks for the paronychia to appear after start of therapy, paronychia may take weeks to improve after cessation of EGFR-inhibitor.[3]

TREATMENT OF HAIR CHANGES, HYPERPIGMENTATION AND TELANGIECTASIA

Eyelashes that cause conjunctival irritation by their excessive length can be trimmed. Hypertrichosis is treated with eflornithine cream or by laser epilation.[11]

Sun protection and adequate treatment of acneiform eruption and eczema are most important to avoid subsequent hyperpigmentation. Bleaching creams are not very helpful but camouflage by a beautician helps to correct the skin color. Left untreated, the hyperpigmentation may fade spontaneously over months.[3]

Telangiectasia caused by EGFR-inhibitors will also gradually disappear over months. Therefore electrocoagulation or pulsed dye laser therapy are only rarely applied to accelerate disappearance. Excellent results can also be achieved with camouflage.[14]

TREATMENT OF MUCOSAL CHANGES

Xerophtalmia, conjunctivitis and blepharitis can be managed with artificial tears, trimming of the eyelashes, topical antibiotics and topical corticosteroids (eye drops or ointment). When superinfection with *S. aureus* occurs, a swab is taken and an oral anti-staphylococcal antibiotic can be added. Refractory cases should be sent to an ophtalmologist as complications such as corneal ulcers may occur.[5]

Tetracycline or antiseptic mouthwash alleviates stomatitis symptoms. For aphtous ulcers of the mouth, topical steroids or anaesthetics can be used.[11]

Dryness of the nose or the vagina is responding fairly well to lubrificants or ointments containing an antibiotic or antiseptic.[11]

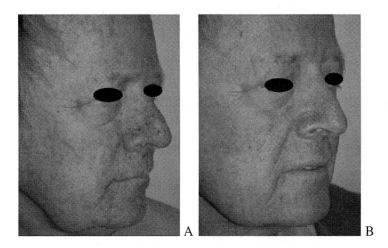

Figure 1. A/ Grade 3 acneiform eruption in a 60-year-old patient with metastatic non-small cell lung cancer receiving erlotinib 150 mg qd since 14 days. Note the numerous pustules on the nose, chin and cheeks. B/ While continuing erlotinib 150 mg qd, patient was treated with saline compresses (twice a day 15 minutes), topical metronidazole 2% cream several times a day and oral minocycline 200 mg qd. Treatment result after 2 weeks is shown with disappearance of the majority of pustules. Metronidazole cream was continued, minocycline dose was lowered to 100 mg qd and compresses were stopped.

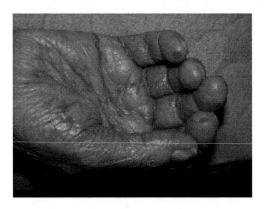

Figure 2. Xerosis, beginning eczema of the hands and fingertip fissures in a patient receiving cetuximab for colorectal cancer since 5 months.

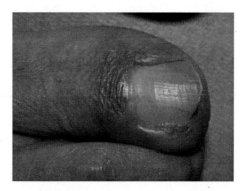

Figure 3. Paronychia and pyogenic granuloma of the big toe in a patient on cetuximab since 4 months for colorectal cancer.

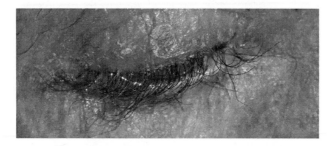

Figure 4. Trichomegaly of the eyelashes and blepharitis in a colorectal cancer patient receiving cetuximab for 6 months.

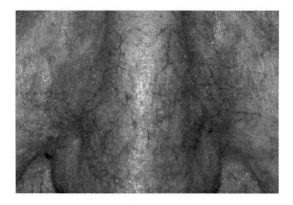

Figure 5. Telangiectasia of the nose in a patient receiving cetuximab for 3 months for colorectal cancer.

CONCLUSION

Despite the absence of evidence-based guidelines, the vast majority of patients experiencing EGFR-inhibitor-induced skin toxicity are easily managed without dose adjustment or interruption of the EGFR-inhibitor. Topical metronidazole and oral minocycline are the mainstay of treatment of acneiform eruption. Frequent use of emollients is the basis to control xerosis and to prevent development of eczema or fissures. Sun protection is advized to all patients.

LEARNING POINTS

- Cancer patients on EGFR-inhibitors are very likely to develop acneiform eruption, skin xerosis, paronychia, hair changes, hyperpigmentation, telangiectasia and/or mucosal changes.
- EGFR-inhibitor skin toxicity has a marked impact on quality of life. Hence, supportive dermatologic care while continuing the EGFR-inhibitor is indispensable.
- General measures include sun protection (to prevent acneiform eruption and hyperpigmentation), use of emollients, bath/shower oil and lukewarm water for hygiene (to prevent xerosis and fissures).
- Acneiform eruption is treated with topical metronidazole ± minocycline 100 mg qd. In case of grade 3 reaction minocycline dose is doubled and saline compresses are added.
- Cefuroxim axetil 500 mg bid is added for *Staphylococcus aureus* superinfection
- Topical or oral corticosteroids or retinoids are avoided because of their unfavourable side effect profile.
- Settled paronychia is hard to treat and does not benefit from surgery. Antiseptic soaks and a steroid paste may alleviate symptoms.

Table 1. Simplified treatment recommendations for the main EGFR-inhibitor-induced skin toxicities

Type of skin toxicity	Treatment recommendation
	General measures: - sun protection - lukewarm water, bath/shower oil for hygiene - emollients on hands and limbs

Acneiform eruption	Mild: metronidazole cream bid
	Moderate: metronidazole cream bid
	                  minocycline 100 mg qd
	Severe: saline compresses 15 minutes bid
	                  metronidazole cream up to 5 times daily
	                  minocycline 200 mg qd
	                  Consider dose adjustment or interruption EGFR
	                  inhibitor when lack of response
	
	Add cetirizine 10 mg qd for itch
	Add cefuroxim axetil 500 mg bid for S. aureus superinfection

Xerosis Eczema Fissures	Emollients Weak topical corticosteroids Propylenegycol 50% in water 30 minutes under occlusion qd salicylic acid 10% ointment qd
Paronychia	Antiseptic soaks bid Paste containing potent steroid, antiseptic and antifungal bid

REFERENCES

[1]   Johnston JB, Navaratnam S, Pitz MW, Maniate JM, Wiechec E, Baust H, Gingerich J, Skliris GP, Murphy LC, Los M. Targeting the EGFR pathway for cancer therapy. *Curr Med Chem* 2006;13:3483-92.

[2]   Busam KJ, Capodieci P, Motzer R, Kiehn T, Phelan D, Halpern AC. Cutaneous side-effects in cancer patients treated with the antiepidermal growth factor receptor antibody C225. *Br J Dermatol* 2001;144:1169-76.

[3]   Segaert S, Van Cutsem E. Clinical signs, pathophysiology and management of skin toxicity during therapy with epidermal growth factor receptor inhibitors. *Ann Oncol* 2005;16:1425-33.

[4]   Lacouture ME. Mechanisms of cutaneous toxicities to EGFR inhibitors. *Nat Rev Cancer* 2006;6:803-12.

[5]   Melichar B, Nemcova I. Eye complications of cetuximab therapy. *Eur J Cancer Care* 2007;16:439-43.

[6]   Perez-Soler R, Saltz L. Cutaneous adverse effects with HER1/EGFR-targeted agents: Is there a silver lining? *J Clin Oncol* 2005;23:5235-46.

[7]   Van Cutsem E. Challenges in the use of epidermal growth factor receptor inhibitors in colorectal cancer. *Oncologist* 2006;11:1010-17.

[8]   http://ctep.cancer.gov/forms/CTCAEv3.pdf

[9]   Segaert S, Tabernero J, Chosidow O, Dirschka T, Elsner J, Mancini L, Maughan T, Morere JF, Santoro A, Sobrero A, Van Cutsem E, Layton A. The management of skin reactions in cancer patients receiving epidermal growth factor receptor targeted therapies. *J Dtsch Dermatol Ges* 2005;3:599-606.

[10] Hetherington J, Andrews C, Vaynshteyn Y, Fishel R. Managing follicular rash related to chemotherapy and monoclonal antibodies. *Community Oncol* 2007;4:157-62.

[11] Segaert S, Van Cutsem E. Clinical management of EGFRI dermatologic toxicities: the Europe perspective. *Oncology* 2007;11Suppl5:22-6.

[12] Jatoi A, Rowland K, Sloan JA, Gross Hm, Fishkin PA, Kahanic SP, Novotny PJ, Schaefer PL, Johnson DB, Tschetter LK, Loprinzi CL. Tetracycline to prevent epidermal growth factor receptor inhibitor-induced skin rashes. Results of a placebo-controlled trial from the North Central Cancer Treatment Group (N03CB). *Cancer* 2008;13:847-53.

[13] Scope A, Agero ALC, Dusza SW, Myskowski PL, Lieb JA, Saltz L, Kemeny NE, Halpern AC. Randomized double-blind trial of prophylactic oral minocycline and topical tazarotene for cetuximab-associated acne-like eruption. *J Clin Oncol* 2007;25:5390-6.

[14] Robert C, Soria J-C, Spatz A, Le Cesne A, Malka D, Pautier P, Wechsler J, Lhomme C, Escudier B, Boige V, Armand JP, Le Chevalier T. Cutaneous side-effects of kinase inhibitors and blocking antibodies. *Lancet Oncol* 2005;6:491-500.

[15] Lacouture ME, Basti S, Patel J, Benson III A. The SERIES clinic: an interdisciplinary approach to the management of toxicities of EGFR inhibitors. *J Support Oncol* 2006;4:236-8.

[16] Guillot B, Bessis D. Aspects cliniques et prise en charge des effets secondaires cutanés des inhibiteurs du récepteur à l'EGF. *Ann Dermatol Venereol* 2006 ;133:1017-20.

[17]   Gutzmer R, Werfel T, Kapp A, Elsner J. Kutane Nebenwirkungen einer EGF-Receptor-Blockade und deren Management. *Hautarzt* 2006;57:509-13.

[18]   Galimont-Collen AFS, Vos LE, Lavrijsen APM, Ouwerkerk J, Gelderblom H. Classification and management of skin, hair, nail and mucosal side-effects of epidermal growth factor receptor (EGFR) inhibitors. *Eur J Cancer* 2007;43:845-51.

[19]   Monti M, Motta S. Clinical management of cutaneous toxicity of anti-EGFR-agents. *Int J Biol Markers* 2007;22:S53-S61.

[20]   Perez-Soler R, Delord JP, Halpern A, Kelly K, Krueger J, Sureda BM, Von Pawel J, Temel J, Siena S, Soulières D, Saltz L, Leyden J. HER1/EGFR inhibitor-associated rash: future directions for management and investigation outcomes from the HER1/EGFR inhibitor rash management forum. *Oncologist* 2005;10:345-56.

[21]   Lynch TJ, Kim ES, Eaby B, Gary J, West DP, Lacouture ME. Epidermal growth factor receptor inhibitor-associated cutaneous toxicities: an evolving paradigm in clinical management. *Oncologist* 2007;12:610-21.

[22]   Luu M, Lai SE, Patel J, Guitart J, Lacouture ME. Photosensitive rash due to the epidermal growth factor receptor inhibitor erlotinib. *Photodermatol Photoimmunol Photomed* 2007;23:42-5.

[23]   Bernier J, Bonner J, Vermorken J, Bensadoun RJ, Dummer R, Giralt J, Kornek G, Hartley A, Mesia R, Robert C, Segaert S, Ang KK. Consensus guidelines for the management of radiation dermatitis and co-existing acne-like rash in patients receiving radiotherapy plus EGFR inhibitors for the treatment of squamous cell carcinoma of the head and neck. *Ann Oncol* 2008;19:142-9.

[24]   Plewig G, Kligman AM (eds). *Acne and rosacea*, 3d ed. Berlin, Springer-Verlag, 2000.

[25]   Perez-Soler R. Topical vitamin K3 (menadione) prevents erlotinib and cetuximab-induced EGFR inhibition in the skin (abstract). *J Clin Oncol 2006 ASCO Annual Meeting Proceedings Part 1* 2006;24:3036.

[26]   Suh K-Y, Kindler HL, Medenica M, Lacouture M. Doxycycline for the treatment of paronychia induced by the epidermal growth factor receptor inhibitor cetuximab. *Br J Dermatol* 2006;154:191-2.

In: Handbook of Skin Care in Cancer Patients
Editors: Pierre Vereecken and Ahmad Awada

ISBN: 978-1-61668-419-8
© 2012 Nova Science Publishers, Inc.

Chapter 3

HOW TO MANAGE HAIR CHANGES IN CANCER PATIENTS

C. Piérard-Franchimont[1], P. Quatresooz[1], A. Rorive[2], G. Piérard[1]

Departments of [1]Dermatopathology, [2]Medical Oncology, University Hospital of Liège, Liège, Belgium

ABSTRACT

Cancer patients under treatment develop quite frequently changes in the density and structure of hair fibres. These alterations mainly result from modifications in the germinative compartment of the hair matrix and in the relationship between melanocytes and trichocytes. As a result hair effluvium and alopecia ensue, but also conversally hypertrichosis and trichomegaly. The hair colour and hair shape are not unfrequently altered. There is no radioprotective agent active against ionizing radiations. In case of short term cytostatic perfusion, scalp hypothermia procedures and tourniquet pressure can help reducing the impact on hair growth. Minoxidil has no preventive effect, but it is susceptible to reduce the severity and duration of cytostatic-induced alopecia. Anyway, any psychological support is always important for the patient. Wearing a wig should be encouraged when needed.

INTRODUCTION

A patient with cancer is possibly affected by hair alteration or loss [1-3]. The process may be focal or widespread, eventually leading to partial, diffuse or total alopecia. The hair loss may be transient but may become definitive. The origin may be one of those recognized for any individual, without any direct or indirect relationship with the cancer or its treatment. However, in some instances, the hair growth and structure are altered by the cancer status. Body hair can also be affected leading to rarefaction and even complete loss [4]. By contrast, other cases show hypertrichosis or hirsutism.

As a result of oncology treatments, alopecia is often transitory but the texture of regrowing hair may be modified. Once induced, hypertrichosis tend to persist. Any pilary change may increase the psychological distress of the affected patients [5]. Not only women but also men can suffer from their modified appearance [6]. Taking in consideration these pilary changes is therefore an important aspect of the patient's management.

HAIR STRUCTURE OF THE SCALP

Terminal hair follicles are found on the scalp, as well as in the axillary and genital areas. They are composed of a portion penetrating deeply into the dermis and the superficial hypodermis, forming a thick hair shaft emerging from the follicle. The infundibulum is the permanent portion of the follicle located above the attachment of the sebaceous duct. Its structure is similar to the epidermis. Smooth muscle fascicules forming the arrector pili extend at an angle between the superficial dermis and a point in the follicular epithelium identified as the bulge. This structure, nearby the hair isthmus, contains a population of hair stem cells able to regenerate a complete follicle after regression of its transient lower portion [7]. The latter structure contains at its proximal end the hair bulb where intense cell proliferation produces the hair shaft. In addition, it contains active melanocytes. The hair shaft is thus composed of trichocytes which are modified keratinocytes. It grows up from the hair matrix being part of the hair bulb covering the dermal papilla. The latter structure contains specialized mesenchymal cells encased within a unique extracellular matrix enriched in glycosaminoglycans.

The hair shaft is a fully keratinized cortex wrapped by the cuticle. A central medulla is variable in size and shape along the hair. It may be continuous, fragmented or absent. The relative proportion of the medulla in the whole hair appears to increase with hair thickness. It reaches a maximum in growing terminal hairs, in which the medulla minor axis represents about 30% of the whole hair shaft minor axis [8]. This proportion appears constant in the terminal hairs.

The volume of the papilla appears to govern the size and shape of hair [9]. Three basic anthropological configurations of hair are recognized. There is no intrinsic difference in the chemical composition between ethnic hair types. The black Negroid hair is woolly and distinctly oval in cross-section showing a high twist ratio. Caucasoid hair is less regular, with a tendency to be oval in cross-section with a variable twist characteristic. It tends to be thinner than Mongoloid hair and exhibits a wide range of colours. The typical Mongoloid hair is cylindrical, thick, straight and black. The alleged relationship between the cross-sectional shape of the hair shaft and the form of the hair, e.g. curly or straight hair, has been challenged. Cell tensegrity depending on the intracytoplasmic cytoskeleton scaffold likely plays a prominent role. A significant degree of polymorphism can occur over time along a given hair shaft, and hair may display mixed conformational characteristics [8].

HAIR CYCLE

Hair growth is under the control of a complex and precise process which is not fully understood [10]. It is a cyclical process, involving synthesis, elongation and, finally, partial regression and shedding of the hair shaft [11]. The hair cycle is made of 3 main stages represented by the anagen, catagen and telogen phases. The anagen phase is the active growth process which normally persists for about 3-6 years or more. It is subdivided into 6 successive substages. The first 5 anagen phases I to V correspond to the hair follicle regeneration, and the last anagen VI phase represents the continuous visible hair growth reaching about 0.35 mm per day. This growth rate is a little bit faster on the vertex than at the periphery of the scalp. Following this growth period, the hair follicle suddenly arrests its proliferative activity and it enters massive apoptosis and a spontaneous involution during the catagen phase. This phase lasts approximately 3 weeks. The next telogen phase is the ultimate period of the hair cycle. It lasts about 3 months during which the hair is fully keratinized. The hair cycle ends with hair shedding. That moment has been called teloptosis [12] or exogen phase [13].

Beginning with the established telogen phase, well before teloptosis, the proliferative activity recovers in the isthmus part of the hair follicle to give rise to the anagen I phase of a new hair cycle [14]. The coordination between the end of a cycle and the surge of the new hair at the scalp surface is not guaranteed. In some instances, the older telogen hair is still present when the new anagen VI hair shows up. Two hairs are then emerging from a single acroinfundibulum. In other circumstances, teloptosis has occurred before the next hair has reached the anagen VI stage. Thus, during that period, the hair follicle appears empty at the clinical inspection. The latency period [15] during which a visible hair is absent corresponds to the hair eclipse phenomenon [16]. Whether this hair eclipse phenomenon represents or not a specific hair cycle phase tentatively called kenogen [17] is a matter of debate [16].

HAIR SHEDDING AND ALOPECIA

Any hair cycle disturbance affecting many follicles may be perceived as an increased hair shedding called effluvium. The process may be reversible or lead to hair loss corresponding to alopecia [18]. Two main biological mechanisms are possible. The hair cycle can be altered by a reduction of the growth period. This condition results in an increased proportion of telogen hairs. As another option, the hair cycle may be altered by the partial or complete inhibition of the anagen phase leading to the appearance of dystrophic hairs [14]. These hairs are lost without evolving through the catagen and telogen phases. Characteristically, subjects are far more concerned about increased hair shedding than the observer looking for alopecia. Several types of effluvium are described in dermatology. They are termed according to the stage of the hair cycle when the shaft is expelled [14, 19-21].

As the damage affecting the matrix can be of variable intensity, the final damage can be expressed by 3 distinct modalities which are called telogen effluvium, dystrophic anagen effluvium and mixed type of effluvium associating the aspects of both telogen and dystrophic types.

Hair shedding is not synonymous with progressive baldness. In fact, it is debatable to what extent telogen effluvium whether sporadic or chronic represents a pathway into alopecia or a self-limiting moult without any consequence for long-term hair density [20, 21]. Telogen alopecia is defined by the premature arrest of hair growth with passage in catagen and telogen phases. This leads to a reduction in the proportion of hairs in the anagen VI phase [18]. Teloptosis occurs about 2 months after the initiation of the process [12]. Anyway, diffuse hair thinning secondary to telogen effluvium may develop. In this case, the proportion of telogen hair is often excessive on the scalp, but it may also decrease when early teloptosis is operative [12, 20]. It is also possible that the emergence of new anagen VI hairs at the skin surface is delayed, giving rise to the hair eclipse phenomenon [16].

Dystrophic anagen effluvium and alopecia are characterized by the presence in excess (above 2%) of hairs in anagen dystrophic phase. This condition is often the clue for an acute and extensive alopecia.

Another cause of alopecia deals with a poor quality of the hair shaft. The defect is rarely congenital, but more often acquired, including the development of brittle hair. Malnutrition observed in some cancer patients could be responsible for such a condition.

MAIN CAUSES OF ALOPECIA IN CANCER PATIENTS

Post Surgical Alopecia

Any surgical intervention on the scalp can be responsible for hair loss or destruction of hair follicles. In some instances, this condition results from the surgical removal of a large skin neoplasm. The resulting post-surgical alopecia is limited to the surgical intervention, and it commonly proves to be permanent. The treatment relies on hair grafting or repair following tissue expansion.

A different condition is represented by alopecia areata secondary to the surgical stress [22]. In such instance, the trichogram reveals a high proportion of telogen hairs with a number of "exclamation-mark" hairs. Alopecia areata must be distinguished from the patchy alopecia induced by some metastases to the scalp [23].

Post Radiotherapy Alopecia

Scalp is irradiated in a number of cancer-related conditions. Radiotherapy may target some cutaneous neoplasms. However, in most instances, a primitive or metastatic neoplasm is targeted in the brain. A post irradiation alopecia is possible depending on the nature and field of irradiation, as well as on the delivered dose [24]. It is often transitory, but it may be permanent. A trichogram reveals dystrophic aspects of anagen hairs. In some instances, radiotherapy induces the so-called erosive pustular dermatosis [25].

When the irradiation is palliative in case of brain metastasis, alopecia is not of prime concern. The situation is different when cure of the neoplasm is expected. There is no means of prevention for post radiotherapy alopecia [26]. Surgery can be proposed for permanent circumscribed alopecia.

Chemotherapy-Induced Alopecia

Cells of the hair matrix can be targeted by cytostatics [11, 27, 28] similarly to other tissues characterized by a high cell turnover. Thus chemotherapy represents the most frequent cause of alopecia in cancer patients. This adverse event is known and dread by many patients. The type of alopecia depends on the nature, dosage and modality of drug administration, as well as on various associations with other drugs. In addition, the individual susceptibility of the patient to the drug is important to consider. The caveolin-1 expression in multipotent cells of hair follicles might be involved in hair resistance to chemotherapy [29]. Anyway chemotherapy-induced alopecia is largely predictable when drugs are administered according to well defined protocols.

The molecular mechanisms responsible for chemotherapy-induced alopecia remain in part unsettled in man. Indeed adequate research models are lacking and animal models are not satisfactory [30]. Quite recently the effects of a metabolite of cyclophosphamide were studied in culture after microdissection of human hair follicles in anagen VI phase [31]. The dystrophic aspects similar to the in vivo situation were reproduced. Keratinocytes and melanocytes of the hair matrix were altered while fibroblasts of the hair papilla remained almost unaffected. The hair matrix became atrophic, the hair shaft narrowed, and the inner and outer hair sheaths partly vanished. Overexpression of p53 protein [27, 32, 33], DNA oxidation and massive apoptosis lead to early regression of the hair follicle (catagen phase, shortening of the telogen phase) or to a complete dystrophic hair follicle (prolonged anagen dystrophic phase). In the former condition, the hair follicles can quite rapidly recover a normal function. In the other condition, the hair cycle recovers more slowly. The hair melanocytes in close contact with the matricial keratinocytes stop the normal production and transfer of melanosomes. Pigmentary incontinence occurs in the perifollicular connective tissue [31].

The anagen dystrophic effluvium and alopecia are frequently reported with cytarabine and occurs in 1-10% of patient [33]. Such an adverse effect usually begins 2-4 weeks after institution of therapy. Alopecia is common in 80% or more patients receiving epirubicine and any taxane [34] but is only rarely caused by gemcitabine. Vinca alkaloids cause alopecia in 20-70% of patient exposed [33, 35], as does etoposide in about two-thirds of patients [36, 37]. The camptothecins and bleomycin also induce alopecia in about 50% of patients [33, 38]. Liposomal delivery of the anthracyclines has been associated with less toxicity including minimal or no alopecia [39]. Dactinomycin has also been reported as a cause of alopecia [40, 41].

The severity of alopecia can be roughly graded according to criteria from the World Health Organization (WHO) or the National Cancer Institute (NCI) (Tables 1, 2). There are other more precise quantitative assessments that can be used in cancer patients [18]. They are listed in Table 3.

The duration of alopecia is variable and influenced by the nature of the chemotherapeutic agent. It is almost always reversible after stopping treatment, with often a lag time of a few weeks after perfusion. Repeating cures is obviously an aggravating factor. Failure of hair regrowth was observed after administration of paclitaxel, docetaxel and aromatase inhibitors as well as after pulse therapy by busulfan [42, 43].

Table 1. Alopecia grading according to WHO

Grade	Aspect
0	Absence of alopecia
1	Mild hair shedding
2	Moderate hair shedding, plaque alopecia
3	Reversible total alopecia
4	Permanent total alopecia

Table 2. Alopecia grading according to NCI

Grade	Aspect
O	Absence of alopecia
T	Partial alopecia
U	Total alopecia
V	Total loss of pilosity

Table 3. Scoring methods for alopecia grading

- Regional hair pattern
- Hair density and part width
- Contrasting felt examination
- Daily hair counts
- Hair pull test
- Hair feathering test
- Quantitative photography
- Hair pluck trichogram
- Hair growth window
- Phototrichogram and videotrichogram
- Tractio-phototrichogram
- Hair weighing

In the majority of cases, cytostatic-induced alopecia is associated with a modification in hair texture [44]. The shape and color of hair shafts can be modified. A trichogram reveals the aspects of any type of alopecia including telogen, dystrophic anagen or mixed pattern [18].

Hair and EGFR-Targeted Therapies

Basic knowledge in oncogenesis has dramatically improved in the last decade providing more recently new drugs for cancer treatment. Some of the new targeted antineoplastic compounds act by inhibiting the epidermis growth factor receptor (EGFR) and its tyrosine kinase transduction pathway involving one or more than one proteins involved in tumor growth and cancer progression [45]. This pharmacological effect is the result of monoclonal or small molecule action which are also responsible for cutaneous adverse effects [45-49] including alterations in hair growth resulting in alopecia. The constellation of findings has been referred to as the PRIDE syndrome, an acronym for papulopustules and/or paronychia, regulatory abnormalities of hair growth, itching, and dryness due to epidermal growth factor receptor inhibitors [47]. Hypersensitivity reactions manifested by a rash, possibly accompanied by anaphylaxis and death, have also been reported [45].

Hair growth is slower and the hair shafts become thinner, brittle and curly [50]. An aspect reminiscent of androgenetic alopecia has been described [51]. A follicular pustular eruption is common [52, 53]. The folliculocentric nature of these adverse reactions is probably due to the presence of EGFR in the outer root sheath cells of hair. The EGFR-ligand system has an essential role in regulation of the hair cycle, as activation of EGFR stimulates transition from anagen to catagen [52, 54].

Other Drugs Responsible For Alopecia

High dose corticosteroids are responsible for occasional telogen effluviums. The selective modulators of the estrogen receptors such as tamoxifene and aromatase inhibitors induce an androgenic type of alopecia.

Interferons induce alopecia in about 50% of cases [55]. It consists in a telogen effluvium which develop after 3 to 4 months of treatment. The severity is variable. The alopecia may be reversible, even when treatment is sustained. Interferons may also induce or aggravate autoimmune disorders such as alopecia areata [56]. Other cytokines like interleukin 2 are also responsible for alopecia [57].

The anti-angiogenic drug sorafenib may also be responsible for alopecia [58, 59].

OTHER HAIR CHANGES

A variety of hair changes occur in some cancer patients including otherwise unidentified hair changes (65%), canitia (gray hair) (40%), repigmented hairs (20%), twisted and curled hairs (35%). Interferon and sunitinib are responsible for canitia in 18% and 30%, respectively of patients [58]. Skin and hair depigmentation is typically present during imatinib [60]. This effect is related to the presence of KIT receptors on melanocytes. Curled hair has been found during acitretin treatment [61].

Dandruff-associated alopecia [62] does not appear to be influenced by cancer therapy. Similarly, alopecia related to tinea capitis is not reported to be more frequent in these patients [63].

Table 4. Hair modifications following chemotherapy

Hair alterations	Frequency (%)
Altered aspect	64
Canitia	40
Repigmented hair	20
Twisted hair	35

Table 5. Alopecia risk according to the nature of chemotherapy

Major risk	Moderate risk	Minor risk
cpt-11	actinomycine D	bleomycin
cyclophosphamide	5-fluorouracile	carboplatine
docétaxel	hydroxyurea	cisplatine
doxorubicine	methotrexate	melphalan
epirubicine	mitoxantrone	thiotepa
etoposide	procarbazine	
ifosfamide	vinblastine	
paclitaxel	vincristine	
topotecan	vinorelbine	

HYPERTRICHOSIS

Hypertrichoses represent another consequence of a disturbed hair cycle. In this case, the anagen phase is extended and the catagen phase is retarded. A delayed teloptosis is another possible cause. The major hypertrichoses cause esthetic problems which are as troublesome as alopecia, particularly in women.

Acquired hypertrichosis lanuginosa may represent a paraneoplastic manifestation [64]. In this case, it affects more frequently women than men. Colorectal carcinomas, as well as lung and breast neoplasias are commonly found. Hypertrichosis possibily precede the disclosure of the neoplasm and it represents a poor prognostic factor because it often accompanies a metastatic neoplasia. The pathogeny is not yet elucidated. It is possible that some growth factors released by the neoplasm boost the hair follicle. Among others, the role of the fibroblast growth factor (FGF) and β-catenin has been raised.

Hirsutism can also accompany ovarian tumours or develop during treatment of breast cancer by tamoxifen or aromatase inhibitors. Some other treatments are also at the origin of diffuse hypertrichosis such as glucocorticosteroids and interferon.

Some hair follicles react in a particular way. This is the case in response to anti-EGFR compounds, either monoclonal antibodies [65] or tyrosine kinase inhibitors [66, 67]. Facial hypertrichosis has been reported [68]. These drugs induce trichomegaly of the eyebrows and eyelashes in many patients [48, 69-71]. Terminal hair development at the tip of the nose was reported in a patient receiving genfitinib for a metastatic lung carcinoma [72]. Eyelash and eyebrow trichomelagy has also been induced by interferon α2a [73].

MANAGEMENT OF HAIR CHANGES IN CANCER PATIENTS

The psychological impact of alopecia is important to consider for the patient [5, 6, 74]. The patient must be aware of and feel at ease about the evolution of the alopecia. All the relevant cosmetic armamentum should be used to minimize the esthetic prejudice. Wearing a wig should be encouraged when needed. It is in part reimbursed by the Social Security in Belgium.

Several modalities have been evaluated to prevent alopecia both in humans and in animal models, including hypothermia and tourniquet pressure. Cooling the scalp to at least 24°C has been advocated in order to prevent or decrease the severity of alopecia in patients receiving short duration intravenous cytostatic perfusions [75-77]. The aim was to get vasoconstriction thus reducing the amount of cytostatic drug presented to the scalp and hair follicles. The shorter the cytostatic half-life in the serum, the better the prevention. The benefit is expected provided vasoconstriction is obtained about 5 min before the initiation of treatment and maintained for about 20 min after the arrest of perfusion [78-80]. Hypothermia may also lower the metabolic rate and simultaneously decrease the rate of drug uptake by cooler tissues. This preventive modality is of no help in case of long duration perfusions and oral treatments. Several cooling devices are available ranging from simple ones with limited capacities to more sophisticated structures. Some patients suffer from headache during scalp cooling. Contra-indications encompass hemopathies and skin or skull metastases. Theoretically, scalp cooling could favor the development of such metastases.

Tourniquet pressure, applied like a headband around the scalp and ranging from 30 to 50mm Hg above systolic blood pressure, has been suggested to abrogate alopecia [78-80], presumably by temporarily decreasing scalp blood flow.

A series of other chemical prevention trials have been performed in the animal using cyclosporine A [81], EGF, p53 protein inhibitor [27] and parathormone/parathormone related peptide receptor [82]. In particular, ImuVert®, an immunomodulator derived from the bacterium *Serratia marcescens*, has been shown to lessen and delay alopecia caused by cytarabine and by doxorubicin in animal models and human trials [78-80]. Vitamin D3 binds to receptors of hair cells and it affects cell growth. Topical applications of vitamin D3 analogues gave contradictory results in the prevention of cytostatic-induced alopecia [83-86]. In general, chemical prevention failed to provide evidence for convincing clinical efficacy.

Topical minoxidil has no preventive effect, but this compound is susceptible to reduce the severity and duration of cytostatic-induced alopecia [80, 87].

Drug-induced hypertrichosis lanuginosa can slowly regress after stopping the inducer drug. By contrast, terminal hairs found in hirsutism do not usually regress even when the cause is withdrawn. For these patients, new epilatory procedures using laser technology could be helpful [88].

CONCLUSION

Among cutaneous adverse effects experienced by cancer patients, hair changes may be the most distressing. The clinical presentations are varied and often linked to specific therapeutic modalities. They range from increased hair shedding, alopecia, alterations in the shape and colour of the hair shafts and, conversely, to unusual hypertrichosis. Preventive methods are limited and quite often disappointing. Psychological support is always important for the patient.

REFERENCES

[1]   Dorr VJ. A practitioner's guide to cancer related alopecia. *Semin Oncol* 1998, 25, 562-570.

[2]   Piérard GE, Paquet P, Piérard-Franchimont C, Rorive A, Quatresooz P. Réactions cutanées indésirables à la chimiothérapie et leurs traitements. *Rev Med Liège* 2007, 62, 457-462.

[3]   Hinds G, Thomas VD. Malignancy and cancer treatment-related hair and nail changes. *Dermatol Clin* 2008, 26, 59-68.

[4]   Velez N, Khera P, English JC. Eyebrow loss : clinical review. *Am J Clin Dermatol* 2007, 8, 337-346.

[5]   Wagner L, Bye GM. Body image and patients experiencing alopecia as a result of cancer chemotherapy. *Cancer Nurs* 1979, 2, 365-369.

[6]   Hilton S, Hunt K, Emslie C, Salinas M, Ziebland S. Have men been overlooked? A comparison of young men and women's experiences of chemotherapy induced alopecia. *Psychooncology* 2008, 17, 77-83.

[7]   Lavker RM, Miller S, Wilson C, Cotsarelis G, Wei ZG, Yang JS, Sun TT. Hair follicle stem cells: their location, role in hair cycle and involvement in skin tumor formation. *J Invest Dermatol* 1993, 101, 16S-26S.

[8]   Hutchinson PE, Thompson JR. The size and form of the medulla of human scalp hair is regulated by the hair cycle and cross-sectional size of the hair shaft. *Br J Dermatol,* 1999, 140, 438-445.

[9]   Elliot K, Stephenson TJ, Messenger AG. Differences in hair follicle dermal papilla volume are due to extracellular matrix volume and cell number: implications for the control of hair follicle size and androgen responses. *J Invest Dermatol,* 1999, 113, 873-877.

[10]   Stenn KS, Nixon AJ, Jahoda CAB, McKay IA, Paus R. What controls hair follicle cycling? *Exp Dermatol* 1999, 8, 229-236.

[11]   Piérard-Franchimont C, Piérard GE. Comment j'explore .. .une perte de cheveux chez un patient cancéreux. *Rev Med Liège* 2004, 9, 525-529.

[12]   Piérard-Franchimont C, Piérard GE. Teloptosis, a turning point in hair shedding biorythms. *Dermatology,* 2001, 203, 115-117.

[13]   Milner Y, Sudnik J, Filippi M, Kizoulis M, Kashgarian M, Stenn K. Exogen, the shedding phase of the hair cycle growth cycle: characterization of a mouse model. *J Invet Dermatol* 2002, 119, 639-644.

[14]   Piérard-Franchimont C, Piérard GE. A propos du follicule pileux et du cycle pilaire: considérations récentes. *Rev Med Liège* 1997, 52, 671-674.

[15]   Courtois M, Loussouarn G, Hourseau C, Grollier JF. Hair cycle and alopecia. *Skin Pharmacol* 1994, 7, 84-89.

[16]   Piérard-Franchimont C, Petit L, Loussouarn G, et al. The hair eclipse phenomenon : sharpening the focus on the hair cycle chronobiology. *Int J Cosmet Sci,* 2003, 25, 295-299.

[17]   Rebora A, Guarrera M. Kenogen: a new phase of the hair cycle? *Dermatology,* 2002, 205, 108-110.

[18] Piérard GE, Piérard-Franchimont C, Marks R, et al. EEMCO guidance for the assessment of hair shedding and alopecia. *Skin Pharmacol Physiol* 2004, 17, 98-110.

[19] Price V, Gummer C. Loose anagen syndrome. *J Am Acad Dermatol* 1989, 20, 249-256.

[20] Headington JE. Telogen effluvium: new concepts and review. *Arch Dermatol* 1993, 29, 56-63.

[21] Whiting DA. Chronic telogen effluvium: increased scalp hair shedding in middle aged women. *J Am Acad Dermatol* 1996, 35, 898-906.

[22] Piérard-Franchimont C, Piérard GE. Paroxysmal reactions of the scalp. *Rev Med Liège,* 2004, 59, 180-185.

[23] Quatresooz P, Piérard-Franchimont C, Arrese JE, Rorive A, Piérard GE. *Comment j'explore... une métastase cutanée. Qui es-tu? d'où viens-tu?* Rev Med Liège 2008, 63, 559-563.

[24] Quatresooz P, Hermanns-Lê T, Piérard GE. *Spectre anatomo-clinique des lésions cutanées radio-induites.* Skin 2008, 11, 108-111.

[25] Trüeb RM, Krasovec M. Erosive pustular dermatosis of the scalp following radiation therapy for solar keratoses. *Br J Dermatol* 1999, 141, 763-765.

[26] Henry F, Xhauflaire-Uhoda E, Piérard GE. *Prévention et traitement des radiodermites.* Skin 11, 140-143, 2008.

[27] Botchkarev VA, Komarova EA, Siebenhaar F et al. p53 is essential for chemotherapy-induced hair loss. *Cancer Res,* 2000, 60, 5002-5006.

[28] Piérard-Franchimont C, Quatresooz P, Berardesca E, Plomteux G, Piérard GE. Environmental hazards and the skin. E*ur J Dermatol* 2006, 16, 322-324.

[29] Selleri S, Arnaboldi F, Palazzo M, Hussein U, Balsari A, Rumio C. Caveolin-1 is expressed on multipotent cells of hair follicles and might be involved in their resistance to chemotherapy. *Br J Dermatol,* 2005, 153, 506-513.

[30] Hendricx S, Handjiski B, Peters EMJ, Paus R. A guide to assessing damage response pathways of the hair follicle: lessons from cyclosphamide-induced alopecia in mice. *J Invest Dermatol* 2005, 125, 42-51.

[31] Bodo E, Tobin DJ, Kamenisch Y, Biro T, Berneburg M, Funk W, Paus R. Dissecting the impact of chemotherapy on the human hair follicle: a pragmatic in vitro assay for studying the pathogenesis and potential management of hair follicle dystrophy. *Am J Pathol* 2007, 171, 1153-1167.

[32] Botchkarev VA. Molecular mechanisms of chemotherapy-induced hair loss. *J Invest Dermatol* 2003, 8, 72-75.

[33] Litt JZ. *Drug eruption reference manual.* 9th ed New York: Parthenon Publishing Group Inc, 2003.

[34] Lombardi D, Crivellari D, Scuderi C, et al. Long-term, weekly one-hour infusion of paclitaxel in patients with metastatic breast cancer: a phase II monoinstitutional study. *Tumor,* 2004, 90, 285-288.

[35] Wyatt AJ, Leonard GD, Sachs DL. Cutaneous reactions to chemotherapy and their management. *Am J Clin Dermatol,* 2006, 7, 45-63.

[36] Fontana JA. Radiation recall associated with VP-16-213 therapy. *Cancer Treat Rep,* 1979, 63, 224-225.

[37] Cetkovska P, Pizinger K, Cetkovsky P. High-dose cytosine arabinoside-induced cutaneous reactions. *J Eur Acad Dermatol Venereol,* 2002, 16, 481-485.

[38]   Verschraegen CF, Levy T, Kudelka AP, et al. Phase II study of trinotecan in prior chemotherapy-treated squamous cell carcinoma of the cervix. *J Clin Oncol,* 1997, 15, 625-631.

[39]   Hussein MA, Anderson KC. Role of liposomal anthracyclines in the treatment of multiple myeloma. *Semin Oncol,* 2004, 31, 147-160.

[40]   Blumenreich MS, Woodcock TM, Richman SP, et al. A phase I trial of dactinomycin intravenous infusion in patients with advanced malignancies. *Cancer,* 1985, 56, 256-258.

[41]   Limpongsanurak S. Prophylactic actinomycin D for high-risk complete hydatidiform mole. *J Reprod Med,* 2001, 46, 110-116.

[42]   Tosti A, Piraccini BM, Vincenzi C, Misciali C. Permanent alopecia after busulfan chemotherapy. *Br J Dermatol* 2005, 152, 1056-1058.

[43]   Machado M, Moreb JS, Khan SA. Six cases of permanent alopecia after various conditioning regimens commonly used in hematopoietic stem cell transplantation. *Bone Marrow Transplant* 2007, 40, 979-982.

[44]   Fairlamb DJ. Hair changes following cytotoxic drug induced alopecia. *Postgrad Med J,* 1988, 64, 907-911.

[45]   Agero AL, Dusza SW, Benvenuto-Andrade C, Busam KJ, Myskowki P, Halpern AC. Dermatologic side effects associated with the epidermal growth factor receptor inhibitors. *J Am Acad Dermatol* 2006, 55, 657-670.

[46]   Gallimont-Collen AF, Vos LE, Lavrijsen AP, Ouwerkerk J, Gelderblom H. Classiciation and mangement of skin, hair, nail, and mucosal side effects of epidermal growth factor receptor (EGFR) inhibitors. *Eur J Cancer* 2007, 43, 845-851.

[47]   Lacouture ME, Lai SE. The PRIDE (Papulopustules and/or paronychia, regulatory abnormalities of hair growth, itching, and dryness due to epidermal growth factor receptor inhibitors) syndrome. *Br J Dermatol* 2006, 155, 852-854.

[48]   Deslandres M, Sibaud V, Chevreau C, Delord JP. Effets secondaires cutanés des nouvelles molécules anticancéreuses: focus sur les molécules ciblant les récepteurs tyrosine kinase et le récepteur à l'EGF. Ann Dermatol, *2008, 135, S16-S24.*

[49]   Hermanns JF, Piérard GE, Quatresooz P. Erlotinib-responsive actinic keratoses. *Oncol Rep,* 2007, 18, 581-584.

[50]   Agero AL, Dusza S, Benvenuto-Andrade C, Busam C, Myskowsky P, Halpern A. Dermatologic side effects associated with epidermal growth factor receptor inhibitor. *J Am Acad Dermatol,* 2006, 55, 657-670.

[51]   Robert C, Sona JC, Spatz A, Le Cesne A, Malka D, Pautier P, et al. Cutaneous side-effects of kinase inhibitors and blocking antibodies. *Lancet Oncol,* 2005, 6, 491-500.

[52]   Van Doorn R, Kirtschig G, Scheffer E, Stoof TJ, Giaccone G. Follicular and epidermal alterations in patients treated with ZD1839 (Iressa), an inhibitor of the epidermal growth factor receptor. *Br J Dermatol* 2002, 147, 598-601.

[53]   Graves JE, Jones BF, Lind AC, Heffernan MP. Nonscarring inflammatory alopecia associated with the epidermal growth factor inhibitor gefitinib. *J Am Acad Dermatol* 2006, 55, 349-353.

[54]   Heymann WR. Epidermal growth factor receptor inhibitors and hair. *J Am Acad Dermatol* 2008, 58, 642-643.

[55] Guillot B, Blazquez L, Bessis D, et al. A prospective study of cutaneous adverse events induced by low dose alpha interferon treatment for malignant melanoma. *Dermatology,* 2004, 208, 49-54.

[56] Fattovich G, Giustina G, Favardo S, Ruol A. A survey of adverse events in 11241 patients with chronic viral hepatitis treated with alpha interferon. *J Hepatol,* 1996, 24, 38-47.

[57] Asnis LA, Gaspari AA. Cutaneous reactions to recombinant cytokine therapy. *J Am Acad Dermatol,* 1995, 33, 393-410.

[58] Robert C, Soria JC, Spatz A, et al. Cutaneous side effects of kinase inhibitors and blocking antibodies. *Lancet Oncol,* 2005, 6, 491-500.

[59] Robert C. Cutaneous side effects of antiangiogenic agents. *Bull Cancer,* 2007, 94, S260-S264.

[60] Chan CC, Yao M, Tsai TF. Diffuse depigmentation in a patient with chronic myeloid leukaemia. *J Am Acad Dermatol,* 2006, 54, 738-740.

[61] Clarke JT, Price H, Clarke S, et al. Acquired kinking of the hair caused by acitretin. *J Drugs Dermatol,* 2007, 6, 937-938.

[62] Piérard-Franchimont C, Xhauflaire-Uhoda E, Loussouarn G, Saint-Léger D, Piérard GE. Dandruff-associated smouldering alopecia. A chronobiological assessment over 5 years. *Clin Exp Dermatol* 2006, 31, 23-26.

[63] Quatresooz P, Piérard-Franchimont C, Arrese JE, Piérard GE. Clinicopathologic presentations of dermatomycoses in cancer patients. *J Eur Acad Dermatol Venereol* 2008, 22, 407-417.

[64] Slee PHTJ, van der Waal RIF, Schagen van Leeuwen JH, et al. Paraneoplastic hypertrichosis lanuginose acquisita: uncommon or overlooked? *Br J Dermatol* 2007, 157, 1087-1092.

[65] Kerob D, Dupuy A, Reygagne P, et al. Facial hypertrichosis induced by cetuximab and anti-EGF monoclonal antibody. *Arch Dermatol,* 2006, 142, 1657-1658.

[66] Pascual JC, Banuls J, Belinchon I, Blanes M, Massuti B. Trichomegaly following treatment with gefitinib (ZD1839). *Br J Dermatol* 2004, 151, 1111-1112.

[67] Lane K, Goldstein SM. Erlotinib-associated trichomegaly. *Ophthal Plast Reconstr* 2007, 23, 65-66.

[68] Morse L, Calarese P. EGFR-targeted therapy and related skin toxicity. *Semin Oncol Nurs,* 2006, 22, 152-162.

[69] Zhang G, Bati S, Jampol LM. Acquired trichomegaly and symptomatic external ocular changes in patients receiving epidermal growth factor receptor inhibitors: case reports and review of literature. *Cornea,* 2007, 26, 858-860.

[70] Carser JE, Summers YJ. Trichomegaly of the eyelashes after treatment with erlotinib in non-small cell lung cancer. *J Thorac Oncol,* 2006, 1, 1040-1041.

[71] Roe E, Garcia Muret MP, Marcuello E, Capdevila J, Pallares C, Alomar A. Description and management of cutaneous side effects during cetuximab or erlotinib treatments: a prospective study of 30 patients. *J Am Acad Dermatol,* 2006, 55, 429-437.

[72] Kim SY, Choi HJ, Park HJ, Lee JY, Cho BK. An unusual terminal hair growth on the nose tip associated with gefitinib therapy. *Br J Dermatol* 2007, 156, 1087-1088.

[73] Goksugur N, Karabay O. Eyelash and eyebrow trichomegaly induced by interferon α2a. *Clin Exp Dermatol,* 2007, 32, 583-584.

[74]   Richardson LC, Wang W, Hartzema AG, Wagner S. The role of health-related quality of life in early discontinuation of chemotherapy for breast cancer. *Breast J* 2007; 13: 581-587.

[75]   Ridderheim M, Bjurberg M, Gustavsson A. Scalp hypothermial to prevent chemotherapy-induced alopecia is effective and safe : a pilot study of a new digitalized scalp-cooling system used in 74 patients. *Supp Care Cancer,* 2003, 11, 317-377.

[76]   Grevelman EG, Breed WD. Prevention of chemotherapy induced hair loss by scalp cooling. *Ann Oncol* 2005, 16, 352-358.

[77]   Spaëth D, Rosso N, Clivot L. Prise en charge de l'alopécie des patients atteints de cancer. *Rev Prat* 2006, 56, 2020-2024.

[78]   Hussein AM, Jimenez JJ, McCall CA, et al. Protection from chemotherapy-induced alopecia in a rat model. *Science,* 1990, 249, 1564-1566.

[79]   Hussein AM. Chemotherapy-induced alopecia: new developments. *South Med J,* 1993, 86, 489-496.

[80]   Hussein AM. Protection against cytosine arabinoside-induced alopecia by minoxidil in a rat animal model. *Int J Dermatol,* 1995, 34, 470-473.

[81]   Paus R, Böttge JA, Henz BM, Maurer M. Hair growth control by immunosuppression. *Arch Dermatol Res* 1996, 288, 408-410.

[82]   Peters EMJ, Foitzik K, Paus R, Ray S, Holick MF. A new strategy for modulating chemotherapy-induced alopecia, using PTH-PTHrP receptor agonist and antagonist. *J Invest Dermatol* 2001, 117, 173-178.

[83]   Harmon CS, Nevins TD. Biphasic effect of 1,25-dihydroxyvitamin D3 on human hair follicle growth and hair fiber production in whole-organ cultures. *J Invest Dermatol* 1994, 103, 318-322.

[84]   Billoni N, Gautier B, Mahé YF, Bernard BA. Expression of retinoid nuclear receptor superfamily members in human hair follicles and its implication in hair growth. *Acta Derm Venereol.* 1997, 77, 350-355.

[85]   Chen G, Baechle A, Nevins TD, Oh S, Harmon C, Stacey DW. Protection against cyclophosphamide-induced alopecia and inhibition of mammary tumor growth by topical 1,25-dihydroxyvitamin D3 in mice. *Int J Cancer* 1998, 72, 303-309.

[86]   Hidalgo M, Rinaldi D, Medina G, Griffin T, Turner J, Von Hoff DD. A phase I trial of topical topitriol (calcitriol, 1,25-dihydroxyvitamin D3) to prevent chemotherapy-induced alopecia. *Anticancer Drugs* 1999, 10, 393-395.

[87]   Wang J, Lu Z, Au JL. Protection against chemotherapy induced alopecia. Pharm Res, 2006, 23, 2505-2514.

[88]   Piérard-Franchimont C, Henry F, Paquet P, Piérard GE. Comment je traite… une hypertrichose. *Rev Med Liège* 2003, 58, 605-610.

In: Handbook of Skin Care in Cancer Patients   ISBN: 978-1-61668-419-8
Editors: Pierre Vereecken and Ahmad Awada   © 2012 Nova Science Publishers, Inc.

Chapter 4

NAIL CHANGES IN CANCER PATIENTS: FROM DIAGNOSIS TO MANAGEMENT

Josette André[1,] and Bertrand Richert[2]*

[1]Université Libre de Bruxelles; University Hospitals Saint-Pierre, Brugmann and the
Child University Hospital Reine Fabiola, Brussels, Belgium
[2]Université de Liège; Dermatology Department, University Hospital, Liège; University
Hospital Saint-Pierre, Brussels, Belgium

ABSTRACT

Nail involvement during chemotherapy is common. Because of the kinetic of nail formation, the nail changes appear several weeks after drug intake. They are characterized by the involvement of several nails, rarely all twenty nails, more often on the fingers than on the toes. Clinical presentation depends on the duration and severity of the toxic injury as well as on the nail component involved, and may result in Beau's lines, onychomadesis, longitudinal melanonychia, onycholysis or pyogenic granuloma. The pathogenesis of nail damage is often not fully understood. These side effects disappear upon cessation of the treatment with the offending drug. They however rarely alter the patient's quality of life and do not impose treatment discontinuance, except occasionally when the most recent chemotherapeutic drugs are involved (taxanes and epidermal growth factor receptor (EGFR) inhibitors). Management is very conservative and mostly orientated towards adequate nail care, in order to help the patient overcome these side effects until the chemotherapy is completed.

---
* Correspondence: Dr Josette André, Dermatology Department, Bd de Waterloo, 129, 1000 Brussels, Belgium. Tel:
+ 32 2 535 43 79; Fax: + 32 2 535 43 81; Josette_andre@stpierre-bru.be

INTRODUCTION

Nail involvement during chemotherapy is common. It rarely alters the patient's quality of life and does not impose treatment discontinuance, except occasionally when taxanes and epidermal growth factor receptor (EGFR) inhibitors are involved. However, the drugs currently used in advanced cancers in women such as taxanes, anthracyclines and topotecan, are frequently responsible for nail changes that alter quality of life. In a recent prospective study on 91 advanced cancers in women, 21 patients (23.1%) developed nail changes such as subungual haematoma, onycholysis, leukonychia or nail loss, and 23.8% of patients with nail toxicities reported these side effects as the most unpleasant [1].

Drug-induced nail changes are characterized by the involvement of several nails, rarely all twenty nails, more often on the fingers than on the toes. The clinical presentation of drug-induced nail changes depends on the duration and severity of the toxic injury, as well as on the nail constituent involved: nail matrix, nail bed, periungual tissues and vessels [2]. Repeated cures are responsible for repeated side effects (Beau's lines, transverse white lines i.e).

The investigation of chemotherapy-induced nail changes are hampered by some confounding factors

- Polychemotherapy is a very frequent regimen that makes the isolation or determination of the main culprit drug difficult.
- The regular adjustments of a chemotherapy regimen with the introduction of new molecules may compound the toxicities to the nail apparatus.
- Radiation, surgery, opportunistic infections may adversely affect nail growth [3].
- Nail alterations may be clinically observed only after several months due to the slow growth of the nail plate [4].
- Moreover, clinical descriptions of nail alterations are often inadequate and may lead to misinterpretation.

In the USA, according to the National Cancer Institute (NCI) Common Toxicity Criteria, nail Adverse Events (CTCAE v3) was graded on a scale of 1 to 3 [5].

- Grade 1 – Mild adverse events: discoloration; ridging (koilonychias); pitting.
- Grade 2 – Moderate adverse events: partial or complete loss of nail(s); pain in nailbed(s).
- Grade 3 – Severe adverse events: interfering with activities of daily living.

Grade 3 was added when nail side effects from taxanes were reported [6]. However, it should be noted that the clinical features described in this score do not reflect those typically seen in response to the EGFR inhibitors. Recently, a new adverse event-specific grading scale for EGFR inhibitors was proposed by the MASCC (Multinational Association of Supportive Care in Cancer) skin toxicity study group [6]. This MASCC scale "is more consistent with dermatologist's terminology as it divides nail abnormalities into those of the nailplate, folds, and digit tips and implements classification similar to an established system for nail psoriasis. The expansion of nail abnormality classification allows for grading of onycholysis, periungual erythema and fissures according to their distinct anatomical side"[6]. Amazingly in the CTCAE v4.0 [7], grade 3 for nail adverse events has disappeared. This scale should be improved accordingly.

In this chapter, the normal nail anatomy will be recalled to mind, and the different nail alterations possibly caused by cancer treatments will be described. Nail adverse events caused by taxanes and EGFR inhibitors will be emphazised. Prevention and management of these nail adverse events will be considered.

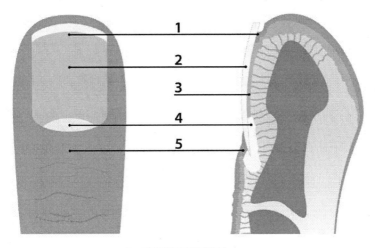

1 - HYPONYCHIUM
2 - NAIL PLATE
3 - NAIL BED
4 - LUNULA/MATRIX
5 - PROXIMAL NAIL FOLD

Figure 1. Basic nail anatomy.

NAIL ANATOMY

The nail plate is a hard keratin plate, set in the soft tissues of the dorsal digital extremity (Figure 1). It stems from the nail matrix located in the proximal part of the nail apparatus. The nail plate and matrix are partly covered by a skin fold called the proximal nail fold. The lunula, a whitish crescent visible at the proximal part of some nails corresponds to the distal, visible part of the matrix. The matrix is a highly proliferative epithelium that differentiates and keratinises, producing the nail plate. The latter grows towards the distal region, sliding along the nail bed to which it adheres closely and from which it only separates at the distal part, called hyponychium. The nail bed epithelium is thin and mainly responsible for its adherence to the nail plate. The nail grows continuously: in 1 month, fingernails grow about 3 mm and toenails about 1mm. This explains why fingernails are more susceptible to anticancer drugs than toenails. A full nail re-growth takes 4 to 6 months for normal fingernails whereas 12 to 18 months is necessary for toenails [9]. Melanocytes are less numerous in the nail apparatus than in the skin. They are mainly located in the matrix. Most of them are dormant and do not produce pigment [10].

NAIL SYMPTOMS

1. *Nail surface alterations.*

   a. *Beau's lines* appear as transverse grooves on the nail plate surface. They are caused by a transient decrease of the mitotic activity of the nail matrix keratinocytes. The depth and width of the groove are respectively related to the degree and duration of the matrix insult. Beau's lines are one of the most common adverse effects of cancer chemotherapeutic agents and reflect their toxicity on the actively dividing nail matrix. They are more commonly observed after short and intensive chemotherapy, specially combined chemotherapy. They may affect all 20 nails but are more frequent on the fingers than on the toes. They appear a few weeks after the beginning of the treatment. Multiple Beau's lines on several nails indicate repetitive treatment cycles (Figure 2) [11].

   b. *Onychomadesis* describes the presence of a transverse whole-thickness sulcus that divides the nail into 2 parts. It represents the extreme degree of a Beau's line and shares the same pathogenesis [11].

   c. *Nail brittleness* presents as a horizontal splitting of the distal nail plate, nail surface peeling, thin nails, resulting in the impossibility to wear long nails (Figure 3). Nail thinning of any origin may be responsible for koilonychia (spoon nail). The impaired general condition observed in cancer patients as well as chemotherapeutic agents are often associated with nail brittleness. It results from mild nail matrix dysfunction.

   d. *Pitting,* as mentioned in grade 1 side effects, is probably not related to chemotherapeutic agents. It represents a focal transient involvement of the proximal matrix as seen in psoriasis and alopecia areata.

2. *Nail colour modifications (chromonychia)*

   a. Brown-black nails *(melanonychia).* Drug-induced melanonychia is due to the activation of matrix melanocytes with incorporation of melanin in the nail plate. It is more frequent in dark-skinned than in fair-skin patients and typically involves several nails [11, 12]. The nail may show 1 or multiple, brown to black longitudinal bands (longitudinal melanonychia) or may be diffusely pigmented (total melanonychia). More rarely, melanocyte activation produces transverse pigmented bands parallel to the lunula, indicating an intermittent production of melanin related to successive courses of chemotherapy (transverse melanonychia). Melanonychia is a common adverse effect of anticancer treatments. Cyclophosphamide, doxorubicin, 5-fluorouracil, bleomycin and hydroxycarbamide (hydroxyurea) [13] (Figure 4) are the most frequently mentioned drugs. Transverse melanonychia may also be secondary to total skin electron beam therapy [14].

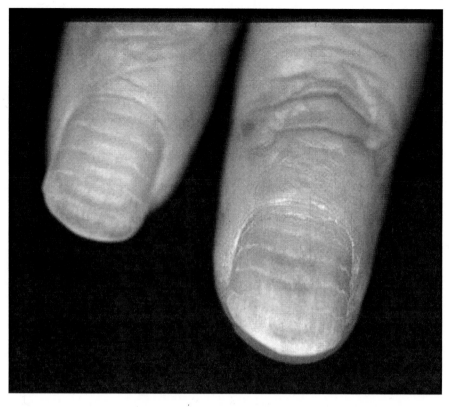

Figure 2. Multiple Beau's lines and transverse true leukonychias (Courtesy O. Correia, Porto, Portugal).

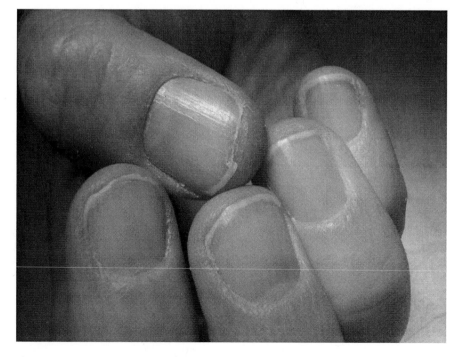

Figure 3. Capecitabine-induced nail brittleness.

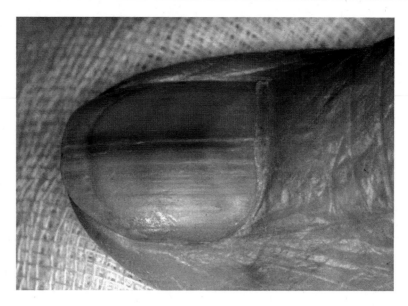

Figure 4. Hydroxyurea-induced longitudinal melanonychia.

b. White nails *(leukonychia)*. True leukonychia results from an insult to the matrix with secondary alteration of the corneocyte filamentous frame or persistence of nuclei in the nail plate. Drug-induced true leukonychia is usually characterized by transverse leukonychia presenting as 1 or by several transverse white opaque bands, 1 to 2 mm wide, that move distally with nail growth (Figure 2). The leukonychia is parallel to the distal lunula. No specific cancer chemotherapeutic drug, combination of drugs or drug class are specific causes of transverse leukonychia, but cyclophosphamide, doxorubicin and vincristine are the most frequently reported offending agents [15]. Apparent leukonychia results from nail bed alterations. It can present as 2 discrete whitish bands (Figure 5), disappearing with pressure and remaining in place while the nail grows. This type of leukonychia was originally described in hypoalbuminemia (Muehrcke's lines) but can also be observed in normo-albuminemic patients [16]. Drug-induced white lines may fade during a pause between chemotherapy cycles. Their physiopathology remains obscure. This was the most common nail change in a series of 30 paediatric patients undergoing chemotherapy [3].

3. *Nail plate Detachment from the Nail bed (Onycholysis)*

Onycholysis describes a separation of the nail plate from the nail bed resulting in the formation of a white-looking space (Figure 6). It can be restricted to the distal part of the nail or be more extensive. Drug-induced onycholysis may be the consequence of a nail bed epithelium injury with secondary epidermolysis and loss of the nail plate adherence. A blue-red onycholysis may also be observed, probably related to the complete destruction of the nail bed epithelium with haemorrhagic blister formation. The latter is very painful. Haemorrhagic onycholysis can also be favoured by thrombocytopenia or anticoagulants. Secondary infections are not rare, giving rise to a yellow or green discoloration. Mitoxantrone and doxorubicin are the drugs most commonly involved in chemotherapy-related onycholysis [17]. Haemorrhagic onycholysis is almost the hallmark of taxane chemotherapy.

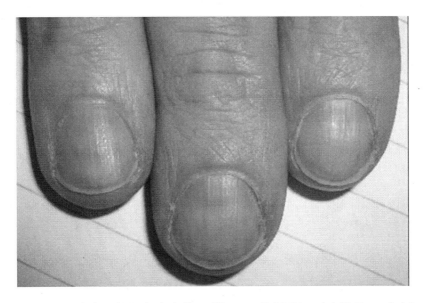

Figure 5. Chemotherapy-induced Muehrcke's lines (Courtesy B.M. Piraccini, Bologna, Italy).

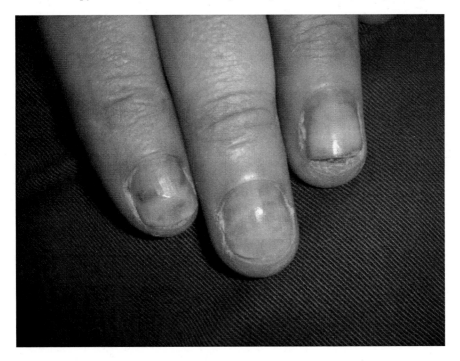

Figure 6. Onycholysis of the ¾ of the nail plate related to taxotere.

4. *Periungual involvement*

Periungual involvement may present as paronychia characterized by erythema, oedema and tenderness in the periungual folds. It can be accompanied by periungual abscesses, granulation tissue (pyogenic granuloma) and ingrown nails. By analogy with retinoids, chemotherapy-induced paronychia and ingrown nails may be a consequence of skin fragility with easier penetration of small nail fragments into the periungual tissues or desquamative dermatitis acting as a foreign body in the lateral nail grooves [18,19,20]. Angiogenic factors can also play a part [21]. Periungual involvement is a common side effect of EGFR inhibitors (see below). Pyogenic granulomas were also reported in association with retinoids, antiretroviral drugs, mitoxantrone [22] and capecitabine [23]. As capecitabine is being increasingly used, clinicians should be aware of this bothering side effect [24]. Recently, pyogenic granulomas have been associated with docetaxel [25,26].

5. *Vessels involvement*

Drugs can also affect the vessels. Subungual splinter haemorrhages are commonly seen with sunitinib and sorafenib, respectively in 30 and 60% of patients. They usually developed in 2 to 4 weeks under the fingernails and less commonly under the toenails. Vascular endothelial growth factor receptor is a target for both sunitinib and sorafenib. It could be involved in the continuous renewal of the delicate spiral capillaries at finger extremities. Blockage of these receptors might hinder physiological repair of traumatised nail bed capillaries [27,28].

TAXANES

Taxanes are microtubule-stabilizing cytotoxic agents. Nail toxicity is one of the most frequent non-haematologic toxicities of docetaxel and often deteriorates a patient's quality of life (QOL) to such extend that it may lead to treatment discontinuation [25]. In a review of the literature, the incidence of patients developing nails changes ranged from 0 to 44 % [2]. More recent studies on a large number of patients found nail side effects in more than 60 % of patients treated with docetaxel, 20 % with paclitaxel [1] and even 88.5 % in patients receiving more than seven cycles [29]. However, these 2 recent studies were using the old version of the NCI CTCAE. It should be noted that a change in Common Toxicity Criteria Grading was suggested by Spazzapan in 2002 in acknowledgment of the severe impact on patient QOL [6]. The version 3.0 of the NCI CTCAE includes grade 3 nail changes (interfering with daily life) whereas version 2 only included ratings up to 2. Amazingly in the CTCAE v4.0 [7], grade 3 for nail adverse events has again disappeared [7]. The previously reported nail change severity was most likely underestimated as a result of a lack of more specific ratings [25]. The largest most recent study using version 3.0, followed 84 patients undergoing chemotherapy with docetaxel for lung cancer. Twenty six percent of patients developed nail changes, including 11 % grade 3. There was no correlation between the development of nail changes and gender. Patients who developed nail changes received a median number of 5 cycles, whereas the respective number for patients without nail changes was 3 cycles. The risk of developing nail changes was significantly higher with the weekly regimen (v thrice weekly docetaxel regimen). The likelihood was 5 % in the first month of treatment, increasing to 60 % at month 6 for weekly docetaxel; whereas the likelihood among the thrice weekly regimen was 0 % for the first month, increasing to only 21 % after 6 months' treatment. This study indicates that more frequent and prolonged exposure to the drug is the most significant risk factor for the development of docetaxel-induced nail changes, regardless of the dose. Most patients developed nail changes after treatment of 3 cycles or more [25]. Also, the use of dose-intensified paclitaxel may induce relevant toxicity to the nail [30]. Patients who received treatment with other kinds of chemotherapy before the treatment with docetaxel were not more prone to developing nail changes [29]. Combination of trastuzumab and docetaxel was responsible for severe nail side effects because of the additive potentially synergistic effect of the two drugs [31].

Nail changes are reported as onycholysis (Figure 6), splinter haemorrhages, haemorrhagic onycholysis (Figure 7) with or without suppuration, development of a typical orange discoloration of the nail plate, and exsudative painful paronychia. Pyogenic granulomas may also occur [25,26]. Subungual hyperkeratosis results from previous exsudative paronychia [32]. Those abnormalities are not serious except for the haemorrhagic onycholysis and the subungual abscesses that can lead to an important morbidity [2]. The latter may result from the neutropeny induced by the chemotherapy, thus enhancing the risk of sepsis [33]. Fingernails are much more often affected than toenails [29].

Various explanations for the pathogenesis of taxane-mediated nail changes have been postulated. It is suggested that direct nail bed toxicity or inhibition of nail bed angiogenesis related to taxane-mediated effects may be the mechanisms leading to onycholysis [34]. A neurogenic mechanism for nail changes is also suggested in the absence of nail change in a denervated hand [35]. The matrix proliferation index in normal nails, calculated by the Ki-67 labelling index, was determined to be 22 % whereas the nail bed measures 0.75% [36]. It therefore appears logical to some authors that drugs such as paclitaxel (which disrupts the cell cycle at the G2 /M phase junction) that inhibit mitosis will mainly affect the nail matrix proliferation, producing abnormalities in the nail plate, whereas drugs such as docetaxel, that act in different phases of the cell cycle, will affect the nail bed and produce onycholysis. For those authors, this assumption is consistent with the high incidence of onycholysis associated with docetaxel and the more frequent reporting of Beau's lines observed with the use of paclitaxel [31]. Another report suggests that paclitaxel, a cremophor EL, acts as a vector. Indeed, it is mentioned that the use of alternative vector formulations are not reported to be associated with nail changes, despite higher dosages in shorter infusion times [37].

Epothilones (ixabepilone), act similarly to taxanes, although they are not structurally related. The first case of nail toxicity was reported after 6 cycles: the patient developed onycholysis and subungual haemorrhagic blisters in the fingernails, which did not impose treatment cessation [38].

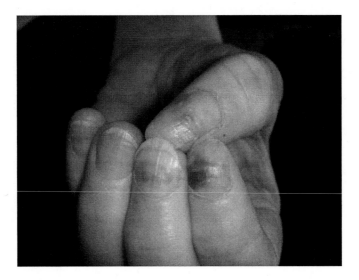

Figure 7. Haemorrhagic onycholysis predominant on the index finger.

EGFR Inhibitors

Two types of EGFR inhibitors can be used: monoclonal antibodies that prevent ligand binding (cetuximab), and small-molecule inhibitors of tyrosine kinase activity (gefinitib and erlotinib). The EGFR inhibitors are generally well tolerated and do not have the severe systemic side effects usually associated with cytotoxic drugs [39]. They however have frequent cutaneous side effects: folliculitis (acneiform eruption), hair modifications, paronychial inflammation and xerosis [28]. Paronychial inflammation was first described with cetuximab in 2001 [40] and 3 years later with gefinitib [19].

Paronychial inflammation, occurring in 10 to 15% of patients treated with cetuximab and gefinitib, is less frequent than acneiform eruption. It typically develops approximately 4 to 8 weeks (sometimes as late as 6 months) after treatment initiation and frequently involves multiples fingers and toes, particularly the great toes and thumbs. It may present as xerosis and a desquamation of the distal digit (Figure 8), acute paronychia, pyogenic granuloma (Figure 9), ingrown nails and periungual abscesses. A secondary infection with *S. aureus* may occur. Lesions tend to wax and wane with continuous therapy; they generally improve with local care, and subside slowly after cessation of EGFR-inhibitor therapy. A correlation between nail toxicity and clinically beneficial response to therapy could not be determined [20,21]. The pathogenesis is not well understood. The epidermal thinning and the nail brittleness induced by these drugs would favour the initial piercing of, or trauma to the periungual skin by the nail plate [20,41]. Also, the development of pyogenic granuloma may be due to angiogenic factors, such as vascular endothelial factor [21].

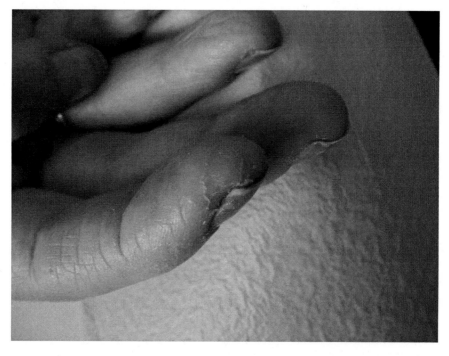

Figure 8. Desquamation of the distal digits with periungual crevice in a patient undergoing EGFR inhibitor treatment.

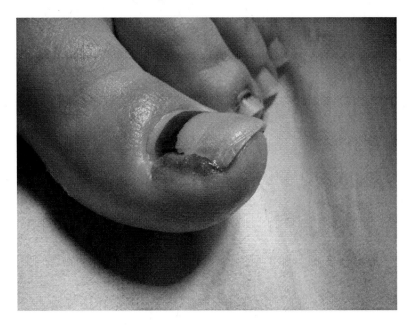

Figure 9. Pyogenic granuloma of the medial nail fold and subacute paronychia associated with EGFR inhibitor. The proximal black pigmentation is a sequela of silver nitrate application.

Management

Beau's lines, onychomadesis, true leukonychia do not require any treatment as they reveal past damage to the nail matrix. They will move distally with nail growth and eventually disappear. In women, leukonychia may be camouflaged with coloured nail polish.

Nail brittleness can be improved by cutting the nails short, reducing contacts with water (patients are advised to ware gloves for house keeping and reduce hand washing), appliance of a nail polish 5 days in 7. Oral intake of biotin (2.5 mg daily) or silicium (12 to 20 mg daily) can also be recommended [42].

When confronted with longitudinal or total melanonychia, nail apparatus melanoma must always be ruled out [43,44]. Usually, it can easily be differentiated from drug-induced melanonychia. Indeed, the latter typically involves several nails while melanoma only involves a single digit. Drug-induced melanonychia does not require any treatment. It is usually reversible. It may however take years to witness the interruption of melanin production by the nail matrix melanocytes after drug cessation [11]. In women, the pigmentation can be camouflaged with coloured nail polish.

Side effects induced by taxanes should be expected, especially if the patient received more than 3 cycles and/or if a weekly schedule is used. A few recommendations should be given to the patient. Some teams recommend the application of a dark nail lacquer in order to prevent sunlight from worsening nail changes [45]. Protection from dirt [29] and atraumatic cleaning of the hands and feet with an antiseptic solution should be recommended in order to minimise the consequences of neutropenia brought on by the chemotherapy. In a study of 49 patients treated with docetaxel, administered every 3 weeks for a median number of 6 cycles, Scotté evaluated the use of a frozen glove (-30°C as used in the cold cap to prevent alopecia) and found that 89 % of patients had grade 0 on the protected hand versus 49 % with nail changes on the unprotected one. Unfortunately, the old and incomplete version of the

National Cancer Institute Common Toxicity criteria was used. However, it was demonstrated that the application of a frozen glove reduced the overall occurrence of nail toxicity from 51% to 11%. The procedure delayed the median time to occurrence of nail toxicity (106 days) compared with 58 days for non-protected group. The device was easily applied, well accepted by most patients and had no major adverse effect [46]. Similarly, the use of a frozen sock significantly reduced the incidence of docetaxel-induced foot nail toxicity [47]. COX2 inhibitors enhance anticancer activity of taxoids. It was recently suggested that they may also prevent adverse side effects of taxanes, including nail changes[48]

In case of painful exsudative onycholysis, only one treatment immediately alleviates the extreme discomfort to the patient: all the onycholytic zones are cut off with adequate nail nippers, thus exposing the swollen and exsudating nail bed where an alcohol-free antiseptic is applied (Figure 10). The nails will grow back normally.

The side effects induced by EGFR inhibitors can be prevented by avoiding trauma to the paronychium (nail biting, tearing of the skin around the nails, overzealous manicure, cutting the nails too short, wearing too tight shoes). Moisturizing creams can be recommended to reduce desquamation of peri-ungual folds. A nail lacquer can be used to harden the nails and prevent nail fragmentation. The patient should be advised to apply some topical steroid associated with an antiseptic as soon as an erythema appears Betamethasone dipropionate, a high potency corticosteroid, twice a day was recommended [49] as well as triamconolone 0.1% and difluprednate ointments [21]. Tetracyclines (doxycycline 100 mg twice daily for 6 weeks) were also prescribed for their anti-inflammatory properties, with inconstant results [49,50]. Secondary infections should be looked for and treated. In case of a staphylococcal secondary infection, flucloxacillin was recommended (500mg three times daily, during 7 days)[41]. Pyogenic granulomas may benefit from silver nitrate applications on a weekly basis. Improvement may rarely require a cessation of the EGFR inhibitor for a short period of time, or a reduction of the dosage. Partial nail avulsion with curettage-coagulation of the granulation tissue should be restricted to the most severe cases, as recurrence is the rule as long as the EGFR inhibitor is maintained [41].

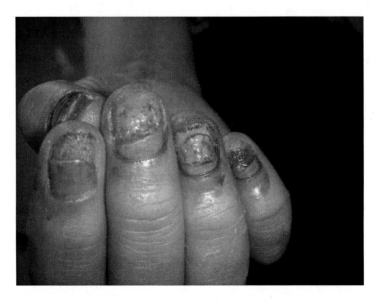

Figure 10. Cutting off the onycholytic areas immediately alleviates pain.

CONCLUSION

Nail alterations in cancer patients are worth being known about. They should be assessed precisely, using the adequate denomination. In most cases, the patients can be reassured as the nail alterations rarely alter their QOL and will eventually disappear without sequelae. More serious nail changes are also described, particularly with taxanes and EGFR inhibitors. The patient must be informed of the possible side effects involving the nails, which ought to be recognized promptly so as to allow adequate management. Treatment cessation is seldom necessary. Further improvement to the CTCAE for nails should be considered.

REFERENCES

[1]   Hackbarth M, Hass N, Fotopoulou Ch et al. Chemotherapy-induced dermatological toxicity: frequencies and impact on quality of life in women's cancers. Results of a prospective study. *Support Care Cancer* 2008; 16: 267-273.

[2]   Minisini AM, Tosti A, Sobrero AF et al. Taxane-induced nail changes: incidence, clinical presentation and outcome. *Ann Oncol* 2003; 14: 333-337.

[3]   Chen W, Yu YS, Liu YH et al. Nail changes associated with chemotherapy in children. *J Eur Acad Dermatol Venereol* 2007; 21: 186-190.

[4]   Piraccini BM, Iorizzo M. Drug reactions affecting the nail unit: diagnosis and management. *Dermatol Clin* 2007; 25: 215-221.

[5]   National Cancer Institute. *Common Terminology Criteria for Adverse Events v3.0* (CTCAE), 2006 August, 9. Available from: URL: http:// ctep.cancer.gov/forms/ CTCAEv3.pdf

[6]   Spazzapan S, Crivellari D, Lombardi D et al. Nail toxicity related to weekly taxanes: an important issue requiring a change in common toxicity criteria grading? *J Clin Oncol* 2002; 20: 4404-4405.

[7]   Lacouture ME, Maitland ML, Segaert S et al. A proposed EGFR inhibitor dermatologic adverse event-specific grading scale from the MASCC skin toxicity study group. *Support Care Cancer* 2010; 18: 509-522.

[8]   National Cancer Institute. *Common Terminology Criteria for Adverse Events v4.0* (CTCAE), 2009 May, 28. Available from: URL: http://evs.nci.nih.gov/ftp1/CTCAE/ CTCAE_4.02_2009-09-15_QuickReference_5x7.pdf

[9]   André J. The Normal Nail. In: M. Paye, A.O. Barel, H.I. Maibach Eds. *Handbook of Cosmetic Science and Technology,* 2^d ed. New York, Taylor & Francis; 2006; pp 89-97.

[10]   Perrin C, Michiels JF, Pisani A et al. Anatomic distribution of melanocytes in normal nail unit: an immuno-histochemical investigation. *Am J Dermatopathol* 1997; 19: 462-467.

[11]   Piraccini BM, Tosti A. Drug-induced nail disorders. Incidence, management and prognosis. Drug Safety 1999; 21: 187-201.

[12]   Ranawaka RR. Patterns of chromonychia during chemotherapy in patients with skin type V and outcome after one year of follow up. Clin Exp Dermatol 2009; 34, e920-e926.

[13]   Aste N, Fumo G, Contu F et al. Nail pigmentation caused by hydroxyurea: report of 9 cases. *J Am Acad Dermatol* 2002; 47: 146-147.

[14] Quinlan KE, Janiga JJ, Baran R et al. Transverse melanonychia secondary to electron beam therapy: a report of 3 cases. *J Am Acad Dermatol* 2005; 53: S112-114.

[15] Chapman S, Cohen PR. Transverse leukonychia in patients receiving cancer chemotherapy. *Southern Med J* 1997; 90: 395-398.

[16] Schwartz RA, Vickermann CE. Muehrcke's lines of the fingernails. *Arch Int Med* 1979;139:242.

[17] Creamer JD, Mortimer PS, Powles TJ. Mitozantrone-induced onycholysis. A series of five cases. *Clin Exp Dermatol* 1995; 20: 459-461.

[18] Baran R. Etretinate and the nails (study of 130 cases) possible mechanisms of some side effects. *Clin Exp Dermatol* 1986; 11: 148-152.

[19] Lee MW, Seo CW, Kim SW et al. Cutaneous side effects in non-small cell lung cancer patients treated with Iressa (ZD1839), an inhibitor of epidermal growth factor. *Acta Derm Venereol* 2004; 84: 23-26.

[20] Fox LP. Nail toxicity associated with epidermal growth factor receptor inhibitor therapy. *J Am Acad Dermatol* 2007; 56: 460-465.

[21] Hu JC, Sadeghi P, Pinter-Brown LC et al. Cutaneous side effects of epidermal growth factor receptor inhibitors: clinical presentation, pathogenesis, and management. *J Am Acad Dermatol* 2007; 56: 317-326.

[22] Freiman A, Bouganim N, O'Brien EA. Case reports: mitozantrone-induced onycholysis associated with subungual abscesses, paronychia, and pyogenic granuloma. *J Drugs Dermatol* 2005; 4: 490-492.

[23] Piguet V, Borradori L. Pyogenic granuloma-like lesions during capecitabine therapy. *Br J Dermatol* 2002; 147: 1270-1271.

[24] Vaccaro M, Barbuzza O, Guarneri F et al. Nail and periungual toxicity following capecitabine therapy. *Br J Clin Pharmacol* 2008; 66: 325-326.

[25] Hong J, Park SH, Choi SH et al. Nail toxicity after treatment with Docetaxel: a prospective analysis in patients with advanced non-small cell lung cancer. *Jpn J Clin Oncol* 2007; 37: 424-428.

[26] Devillers C, Vanhooteghem O, Henrijean A et al. Subungueal abscesses and pyogenic granuloma secondary to docetaxel (taxotere®) therapy. *Clin Exp Dermatol* 2009; 34: 251-252.

[27] Robert C, Faivre S, Raymond E et al. Subungual splinter haemorrhages: a clinical window to inhibition of vascular endothelial growth factor receptors? *Ann Int Med* 2005; 143: 313-314.

[28] Robert C, Soria JC, Spatz A, et al. Cutaneous side-effects of kinase inhibitors and blocking antibodies. *Lancet Oncol* 2005; 6: 491-500.

[29] Winther D, Saunte DM, Knap M et al. Nail changes due to docetaxel-a neglected side effect and nuisance for the patient. *Support Care Cancer* 2007; 15: 1191-1197.

[30] Lüftner D, Flath B, Akrivakis C et al. Dose-intensified weekly paclitaxel induces multiple nail disorders. *Ann Oncol* 1998; 9: 1139-1140.

[31] Alexandrescu DT, Vaillant J, Wiernik PH. Trastuzumab/docetaxel-induced nail dystrophy. *Int J Dermatol* 2006; 45: 1334-1336.

[32] Correia O, Azevedo C, Pinto Ferreira E et al. Nail changes secondary to docetaxel (taxotere). *Dermatology* 1999; 198: 288-290.

[33] Vanhooteghem O, Richert B, Vindevoghel A et al. Subungal abscess: a new ungual side-effect related to docetaxel therapy. *Br J Dermatol* 2000; 143: 462-463.

[34] Vanhooteghem O, André J, Vindevoghel A et al. Docetaxel-induced subungual hemorrhage. *Dermatology* 1997; 194: 419-420.

[35] Wasner G, Hilpert F, Schattschneider J et al. Docetaxel-induced nail changes - a neurogenic mechanism: a case report. *J Neurooncol* 2002; 58: 167-174.

[36] de Berker DAR, Angus B. Proliferative compartments in the normal nail unit. *Br J Dermatol* 1996; 135: 555-559.

[37] Minutilli E, Izzo F, Natoli G et al. Paclitaxel-induced nail changes: possible role of its vehicle (cremophor el). *Eur J Dermatol* 2006; 16: 693-694.

[38] Alimonti A, Nardoni C, Papaldo P et al. Nail disorders in a woman treated with ixabepilone for metastatic breast cancer. *Anticancer Res* 2005; 25: 3531-3532.

[39] Segaert S, Van Cutsem E. Clinical signs, pathophysiology and management of skin toxicity during therapy with epidermal growth factor receptor inhibitors. *Ann Oncol* 2005; 16: 1425-1433.

[40] Busam KJ, Capodieci P, Motzer et al. Cutaneous side-effects in cancer patients treated with the antiepidermal growth factor receptor antibody C225. *Br J Dermatol* 2001; 144: 1169-1176.

[41] Galimont-Collen AFS, Vos LE, Lavrijsen APM et al. Classification and management of skin, hair, nail and mucosal side-effects of epidermal growth factor receptor (EGFR) inhibitors. *Eur J Cancer* 2007; 43: 845-851.

[42] Colombo VE, Gerber F, Bronhofer M et al. Treatment of brittle fingernails and onychoschizia with biotin: scanning electron microscopy. *J Am Acad Dermatol* 1990; 23: 1127-1132.

[43] André J, Lateur N. Pigmented nail disorders. *Dermatol Clin* 2006; 24: 329-339.

[44] Braun RP, Baran R, Le Gal FA et al. Diagnosis and management of nail pigmentations. *J Am Acad Dermatol* 2007; 56: 835-847.

[45] Hussain S, Anderson DN, Salvatti ME et al. Onycholysis as a complication of systemic cancer chemotherapy: report of five cases associated with prolonged weekly paclitaxel therapy and review of the literature. *Cancer* 2000; 88: 2367-2371.

[46] Scotté F, Tourani JM, Banu E et al. Multicenter study of a frozen glove to prevent docetaxel-induced onycholysis and cutaneous toxicity of the hand. *J Clin Oncol* 2005; 23: 4424-4429.

[47] Scotté F, Banu E, Medioni J et al. Matched case-control phase 2 study to evaluate the use of a frozen sock to prevent docetaxel-induced onycholysis and cutaneous toxicity of the foot. *Cancer* 2008; 112: 1625-1631.

[48] Nakamura S, Kajita S, Takagi A et al. Improvement in docetaxel-induced nail changes associated with cyclooxygenase-2 inhibitor treatment. *Clin Exp Dermatol* 2009; 34, e320-e321.

[49] Coquart N, Karam A, Metges J et al. Intérêt de la corticothérapie locale dans le traitement des paronychies aseptiques induites par les inhibiteurs de croissance épidermique. *Ann Dermatol Venereol* 2007; 134: 7S257 (Poster 296).

[50] Shu KY, Kindler HL, Medecina M et al. Doxycycline for the treatment of paronychia induced by the epidermal growth factor receptor inhibitor cetuximab. *Br J Dermatol* 2006; 154: 191-192.

In: Handbook of Skin Care in Cancer Patients   ISBN: 978-1-61668-419-8
Editors: Pierre Vereecken and Ahmad Awada   © 2012 Nova Science Publishers, Inc.

Chapter 5

CANCER AND PHOTOPROTECTION

Christelle Comte, and Bernard Guillot[*]

Dermatology Department, University Hospital of Montpellier,
F34295 Montpellier cedex 5, France

ABSTRACT

Patients undergoing treatment for a cancer don't know which attitude to adopt with the sun. Indeed, some treatments can be very sensitizing and may cause skin burns, even when the exposure occurs before the start of the cure. This chapter attempts to list these treatments. Too much exposure to the sun can also cause skin cancers and patients need to know how to protect themselves. Paradoxically however, sun may also contribute in fighting against the tumoral proliferative process, via synthesis of vitamin D, which is one of the fundamental hormones for our immune system.

1. IS IT NECESSARY TO BE PROTECTED FROM THE SUN WHEN ONE HAS A CANCER? CAN THE SUN CAUSE CANCERS?

Sun and Skin Cancers

It is now a well-known fact that the sun may cause cancers. However, this generality differs somewhat in relation with the type of skin cancer:

Carcinoma

Carcinoma is a cancer of the skin that develops from skin keratinocytes. There are two types of carcinomas: basal cell carcinoma, whose malignity remains strictly local, and

---

[*] For all correspondances : b-guillot@chu-montpellier.fr

squamous cell carcinoma, which can generate remote metastases and whose evolution is systemic like any other cancer.

These carcinomas are generated directly by the sun. They nearly always grow on areas of the body exposed to the sun such as face, cranium, ears, back of the hands, back, scoop-neck…, and occurrence increases the closer one gets to the equator (for subjects with white skin). People with black skin are quite well protected thanks to the large quantity of melanin contained in their skin. The role of acute or chronic occasional or daily exposures is more controversial. However, it seems that there is a connection between squamous cell carcinomas and cumulative quantity of exposure during life, whereas basal cell carcinomas may be caused by excessive exposure and sunstrokes in childhood. [1,2]

Melanoma

Melanomas are skin cancers developed from melanocytic cells (cells synthesizing melanin). Prognosis of these cancers, which are known for developing remote metastasises, is often more serious than in the case of carcinomas. Although the sun plays a role in their occurrence, the major risk factor is not actually the sun but the number of "beauty spots" exceeding 20 and also probably a genetic predisposition. However, the sun can be a cause when the skin has been exposed during childhood and this is especially true of individuals with lightly pigmented skin. Since there is nothing one can do at the present time to modify the genetic component, child photoprotection remains the top priority in the fight against melanoma.

What about Sunbeds?

Sunbeds are ultraviolet A (UVA) lamps. It means that they can have the same effects than sun on skin. They can be responsive of photosensitization of skin when one is in the course of chemotherapy, or radiotherapy, and must be avoid. As for risk of skin cancer: for carcinomas, it has been shown that they can be responsive of basal cell and squamous cell carcinoma. For melanoma risk, as for the sun, the question is more discussed. Several studies showed an increased risk [3], whether other failed to show an increased risk [4]. However, it is probably a risk factor for predisposed people, in particular children and fair skin people, and perhaps for people with particular genetic predisposition.

Sun and other "Internal" Cancers

In recent years, several studies have highlighted the fact that the mortality rate for several cancers depends, in each country, on a North-South latitude gradient [5]: prostate, bladder, esophageal, kidney, pancreatic, rectal, lung, ovary, colon, non-Hodgkin lymphoma, stomach, rectum, corpus uteri, larynx, kidney, and perhaps also melanoma [6,8]. For some cancers, incidence in the USA is about twice as high in the North-West as in the South-East [9] of the country. These differences are even greater beyond latitude 40°. Beyond this latitude, vitamin

D deficiencies are more frequent due to a weaker exposure to sun in general, and to UVB in particular. Hence, the assumed protective role of vitamin D and, by extension, of the sun.

An argument in favour of this assumption is the incidence of second cancers following a diagnosis of skin cancer. It has been noted that, for individuals diagnosed with cutaneous épidermoïd carcinoma, the chances of developing a stomach or colo-rectal cancer are significantly low [9]. For people diagnosed with cutaneous carcinoma in general, the chances of developing a oesophagus, rectum, stomach, or cervix cancer are significantly low. On the other hand, the risk of developing a lip or salivary gland cancer, or a melanoma, is significantly increased. In the case of melanoma, the question may seem paradoxical since in Norway, for example, the incidence is twice as high in the South of the country as in the North, and mortality ratio on the incidence is higher in the North where exposure to UVB is lower. This is also the case in Australia and New Zealand [10]. If the sun is effectively the cause of these observed differences, in terms of public health it will be important for this parameter to be taken into account. As yet, however, the role of UVB and vitamin D is merely a hypothesis in explaining this phenomenon. In addition, an oral supplementation [11] of vitamin D may suffice to attain adequate serum rates of D3 vitamin.

Moreover, for individuals with lightly pigmented skin, photosynthesis of vitamin D occurs in merely a few minutes for an exposure of a small percentage of skin (face and back of the hands) and then reaches a plateau at a sub-erythematogene dose. Prolonged exposure beyond this threshold does not allow storage of additional vitamin D but exposes on the other hand to DNA changes (and consequently to risks of skin cancer) on a linear mode with time [12].

In conclusion, most authors insist on the need for further exploratory studies using instruments providing reliable measurements of radiation effectively received by individuals. It will be necessary to follow these conclusions in the years to come.

2. Is the Sun Dangerous when One Is in the Course of Chemotherapy?

Most chemotherapies do not pose particular problems with the sun. However, some make the skin more sensitive towards the sun and when exposed, all patients suffer from burn or sunstroke of various degrees. More rarely, when exposed to the sun, some patients develop an allergy to certain chemotherapies. This is known as the photoallergy phenomenon.

Definition of Photosensitivity

Phototoxic reaction is common photosensitivity reaction. It can be produced in most individuals given a high enough dose of drug and sufficient light exposure. This photosensitivity reaction is usually evident within 5-20 hours of exposure and resembles an exaggerated sunburn (redness, swelling, blistering, weeping and peeling). The rash is confined to areas exposed to light: face, arms, hands...List of photosensitive chemotherapies is summarized in Table 1.

Nail Impairment

Certain chemotherapies lead to a nail impairment called onycholysis (splitting and separation of the distal part of the nail). The sun would appear to be partly responsible for this process (photo-onycholysis). Indeed, protecting the nails from the sun, use of opaque varnishes, or sun lotions, prevents onycholysis, in particular in the case of anthracyclines and taxanes [21].

Définition of Photoallergy

Photoallergic reaction is much rarer than phototoxic reaction. A photoallergic reaction occurs only in predisposed people. It may have several clinical aspects (eczema, lichenoid eruption...) and may spread beyond areas exposed to light (Table 2).

Table 1. List of photosensitive chemotherapies:

Photosensitive chemotherapies :
Methotrexate [13]
5FU [14]
anthracyclines
- doxorubicine [14]
- farmorubicine [15]
Mitomycine
Cyclophosphamide
Dacarbazine [14]
Procarbazine
Actinomycine D
Vinblastine [16]
Flutamide [17]
Lonidamide [18]
combination of paclitaxel and trastuzumab [19]
Imatinib [20]

Table 2. examples of photoallergic reactions

Drugs	Skin eruptions
fluorouracil derivative (Tegaful) capecitabine	-lichenoid and eczematous eruptions [14, 22] -pellagra [23] -lichenoid eruption [24]
anti EGF recepteur: cetuximab	eczematiform eruptions on photoexposed areas, around eyes, mouth and nose [25]
hydroxyurea	granulomatous eruption [26]
Flutamide	pseudoporphyria [27,28]

Treatment of these Symptoms

- Use cool wet dressings
- Apply topical creams containing corticosteroids, or healing properties
- If the reaction is severe, oral drugs can be prescribed: anti-inflammatory drugs, systemic corticosteroids.
- Following treatment, an adapted photoprotection is necessary (see chapter 5).

3. SHOULD ONE KEEP OUT OF THE SUN FOLLOWING RADIOTHERAPY?

After radiotherapy, patients should keep out of the sun due to the summation of the deleterious effects of ionising and UV radiations. Irradiated areas should therefore not be exposed to the sun during the entire year following radiotherapy in order to avoid the appearance of painful cutaneous reactions.

During chemotherapy, can an old sunstroke or an old "burn" induced by the radiotherapy reappear?

Definition of Photo-recall Phenomenon and Radiation Recall

Photo recall phenomena are well known to occur in patients receiving chemotherapeutic agents after sustaining prior skin damage from radiation therapy or the sun.

Radiation recall is defined as the "recalling" by skin of previous radiation exposure in response to the administration of certain response-inducing drugs [29,30]. The most frequent clinical picture is an erythema sometimes associated with oedema, vesiculation or desquamation, closely limited to the previously irradiated area. Pruritus is common [14]. No exact cause has been documented. More-severe skin reactions may occur more frequently when the period between radiation and the recall-triggering drug is short. The median time between the conclusion of radiation treatment and the occurrence of radiation recall is about 40 days [31]. Most recall reactions have occurred when radiotherapy and chemotherapy are separated by less than 2 months.

Although the precise mechanism of action for this phenomenon is not known, several mechanisms that may lead to the development of radiation recall have been proposed, including changes in vascularization, DNA repair, radiation-impaired epithelial function of stem cells, and increased sensitivity to drugs [28,29].

Which Chemotherapies Can be Responsive?

Four chemotherapies have been documented to be more commonly involved: docetaxel, doxorubicin, gemcitabine, and paclitaxel. However, a lot of cytotoxic agents can be responsive [14]: (Table 3)

How to Avoid it?

Corticosteroids have been suggested to have some protective effects. They should be given following treatment when the phenomenon is noted at the time of the first session.

Concerning methotrexate, the physician must also remember to inform his/her patients that they should avoid exposing themselves to the sun not only after the perfusion but also during the 3 days preceding it.

Table 3. Radiation recall dermatitis–inducing drugs

Drug
Actinomycine [32]
Hydroxyurea [33]
Vinblastine [34]
Doxorubicin [54]
/liposomal doxorubicin [59]
idarubicin [35-37]
epirubicin [38]
Etoposide [39]
Methotrexate [40]
Trimetrexate, edatrexate [41,42]
Tamoxifen [43]
Taxanes [53]
Paclitaxel 44,45]
Docetaxel [46, 56]
Bleomycine [47]
Gemcitabine [48]
Oxiplatine [49]
Dacarbazine [50]
Capecitabine [51]
Interferon alpha 2b [52]
Arsenic trioxyde [55]
Pemetrexed [57]
Hypericin [31]

4. SHOULD ONE KEEP OUT OF THE SUN AFTER SURGERY?

After a surgery, it is better to protect the scar from the sun: indeed, for two years, the scar will change. In the first two month, it will be red and sometimes inflated. About 21 days after the surgery, the skin is continue on the scar, and can be wet: bath are authorized. But, if it is exposed to the sun, it can pigment, and this pigmentation will be permanent. After, the scar become white, and can be exposed. It can take 6 month to 2 years, depending on people. So, until the scar is white, it must be protected by clothes, by dressings, or by a thick lawer of sunscreen, put each 2 hours.

5. HOW TO EFFICIENTLY PROTECT ONESELF FROM THE SUN?

Internal Photoprotection

The aim of internal photoprotection is to protect the individual from the effects of carcinogenesis induced by the sun. As these phenomena are mainly in connection with the generating of "free radicals "or SRO "species reactive oxygenates", the products used are antioxidants such as beta-carotene, vitamins A, C, E, and trace elements: vegetable selenium, zinc, manganese, copper, extracts (flavonoïds, green tea, Polypodium leucotomos. carotenoids: beta-carotene, lycopene) fatty-acids omega-3, Currently, antioxidants have demonstrated their efficiency both in vitro and in animal tests, but there is a lack of scientific evidence of this efficiency in man [60].

Antioxidants can be administered by means of a diet enriched with certain foods, or more simply by ingestion of food compound capsules.

Most orally administered antioxidants have yielded positive results both in vitro and in animal. In the case of man, however, efficiency of antioxidants in the prevention of photo-induced impairment has yet to be established more conclusively.

Foods with high flavonoïd contents are probably the most efficient (along with external photoprotection), but clinical evidence is lacking.

External Photoprotection

Clothing

Clothing constitutes a screen against sun penetration. However, the protection coefficient varies enormously according to the nature, colour and thickness of the fabric [61].

Fabrics providing the best protection include cotton, silk and reflective polyester. Dark coloured clothing is definitely more protective than light coloured clothing but it has the disadvantage of being uncomfortable to wear in summer because of the heat. The coefficient protection from one garment to another can vary from 2 for a polyester dress to over 1,000 for a pair of denim jeans. It should also be noted that wet clothing loses most of its protective capacity [62]. Protecting the face by means of a broad-rimmed hat rather than a cap, which protects neither the ears nor the nape of the neck, is also advisable. UV blocking sunglasses, gloves and scarves should be used as often as possible.

Sunscreens

Although this matter has been the subject of many debates in recent years, the use of a broad spectrum sun lotion (protecting from the UVB and the UVA) would appear to protect against skin cancers. This has been demonstrated for squamous cell carcinomas but not for basal cell carcinomas [63]. Concerning melanomas, the evidence is indirect. Indeed, several studies have shown that the use of sun lotions decreases the number of naevi acquired during childhood [64] and it is a well known fact that a large number of naevi is the first risk factor of melanoma. It is important to consider that the screen applied should not be the cause of a more prolonged solar exposure, which would then increase the risk factor.

The Different Types of Sun Lotions

There are two main types of sun lotions: cream screens, and creams containing chemical filters. Cream screens contain micronized mineral particles (magnesium, titanium, iron, zinc oxides...), which mechanically reflect UV rays. Because of their white colour, cream screens are less cosmetic than filters. They are, however, very effective and stable. Moreover, the occurrence of skin allergy is less frequent with this type of lotion.

Of the many sun filters available on the market, most are combined with a preparation that adds to their intrinsic properties, stability, persistence and UV absorption spectrum. Other substances are sometimes added to the composition of sun lotions in order to combat locally against the harmful effects of UV on the skin. These substances are mostly antioxidants (identical to those used for internal detoxification): vitamins A, C, E, selenium, green tea, lycopenes. . . .

Sun Protection Factor (SPF) and the Way to Use it

SPF numbers on a package can range from as low as 2 to as high as, up to date, 50, or 50+. These numbers refer to the product's ability to screen or block out the sun's burning rays.

The SPF rating is calculated by comparing the amount of time needed to produce a sunburn on protected skin to the amount of time needed to cause a sunburn on unprotected skin. It concerns moreover UVB. But now, sunscreen have to proove a good protection against UVA too, so as UVB/UVA ratio is inferior to 3.

Table 4. Sun protection factors

Low protection	SPF 6-15
Medium protection	SPF 20-25
High protection	SPF 30-50
very high protection	SPF 50 +

The more the skin is white, the more the SPF of sunscreen used must be hight.

But, since those indexes were too complicated to understand for general public, a european commission (september, the 22th, 2006) recommended to simplify the packaging of sunscreens, and to apply new pictograms, and new rule for labelling of sunscreens: there will be only 4 categories (table 4):

CONCLUSION

With the exception of certain chemotherapy and radiotherapy cures during which exposure to the sun is clearly contra-indicated, the advised attitude with respect to the sun is an attitude of moderation: a little sun is beneficial and helps to stimulate the mechanisms that fight against cancer, too much sun can, on the contrary, cause skin cancers. A few minutes of exposure every day whilst avoiding the midday sun is probably beneficial, but should be avoid during cancer treatment.

REFERENCES

[1] Zanetti R, Rosso S, Martinez C, Navarro C, Schraub S, Sancho-Garnier H, et al The multicentre south European study "Helios" I: skin characteristics and sunburns in basal cell and squamous cell carcinoma of the skin. *Br J Cancer* 1996; 73: 1440-6.

[2] Rosso S, Zanetti R, Martinez C, Tormo MJ, Schraub S, Sancho-Garnier H, et al The multicentre south European study "Helios" II: different sun exposure patterns in the aetioogy of basal cell and squamous cell carcinoma of the skin. *Br J Cancer* 1996; 73: 1447-54.

[3] Gallagher RP, Spinelli JJ, Lee TK, Tanning beds, sunlamps, and risk of cutaneous malignant melanoma, *Cancer Epidemiol Biomarkers Prev.* 2005 ;14:562-6.

[4] Bataille V, Boniol M, De Vries E, Severi G, Brandberg Y, Sasieni P, Cuzick J, Eggermont A, Ringborg U, Grivegnée AR, Coebergh JW, Chignol MC, Doré JF, Autier P. A multicentre epidemiological study on sunbed use and cutaneous melanoma in Europe, *Eur J Cancer* 2005;41:2141-9.

[5] Grant WB, An estimate of premature cancer mortality in the U.S. due to inadequate doses of solar ultraviolet-B radiation, *Cancer,* 2002;94:1867-75.

[6] Tuohimaa P, Pukkala E, Scelo G, et al, Does solar exposure, as indicated by the non-melanoma skin cancers, protect from solid cancers: Vitamin D as a possible explanation, *Eur J Cancer* 2007; 43: 1701-12.

[7] Osborne JE, Hutchinson PE, Vitamin D and systemic cancer: is this relevant to malignant melanoma*?*, 2002;147:197-213.

[8] Van der Rhee HJ, de Vries E, Coebergh JW, Does sunlight prevent cancer? A systematic review, *Eur J Cancer* 2006; 42: 2222-32.

[9] Grant WB, A meta-analysis of second cancers after a diagnosis of nonmelanoma skin cancer: additional evidence that solar ultraviolet-B irradiance reduces the risk of internal cancers, *J Steroid Biochem Mol Biol.* 2007;103:668-74.

[10] Moan J, Porojnicu AC, Dahlback A. Ultraviolet radiation and malignant melanoma. *Adv Exp Med Biol.* 2008;624:104-16.

[11] Trivedi DP, Doll R, Khaw KT, Effect of four monthly oral vitamin D3 (cholecalciferol) supplementation on fractures and mortality in men and women living in the community: randomised double blind controlled trial.*BMJ.* 2003;326:469.

[12] Wolpowitz D, Gilchrest BA The vitamin D questions: how much do you need and how should you get it?, *J Am Acad Dermatol.* 2006;54:301-17.

[13] Armstrong RB, Poh-Fitzpatrick MB, Methotrexate and ultraviolet radiation, *Arch Dermatol.* 1982;118:177-8.

[14] Guillot B, Dereure O, Bessis D, Mucocutaneous side effects of antineoplastic chemotherapy, *Expert Opin Drug Saf.* 2004; 3: 579-87.

[15] Balabanova MB, Photoprovoked erythematobullous eruption from farmorubicin, *Contact Dermatitis,* 1994;30:303-4.

[16] Breza TS, Halprin KM, Taylor JR, Photosensitivity reaction to vinblastine, *Arch Dermatol.* 1975;111:1168-70.

[17] Leroy D, Dompmartin A, Szczurko C, Flutamide photosensitivity, *Photodermatol Photoimmunol Photomed.* 1996;12:216-8.

[18]   Battelli T, Manocchi P, Giustini L, Mattioli R, Ginnetti A, De Gregorio M, De Martino C, Silvestrini B. A long-term clinical experience with Lonidamine.*Oncology.* 1984;41:39-47.

[19]   Cohen AD, Mermershtain W, Geffen DB, Schoenfeld N, Mamet R, Cagnano E, Cohen Y, Halevy S, Cutaneous photosensitivity induced by paclitaxel and trastuzumab therapy associated with aberrations in the biosynthesis of porphyrins, *J Dermatolog Treat.* 2005;16:19-21.

[20]   Rousselot P, Larghero J, Raffoux E, Calvo F, Tulliez M, Giraudier S, Rybojad M, Photosensitization in chronic myelogenous leukaemia patients treated with imatinib mesylate, *Br J Haematol.* 2003;120:1091-2.

[21]   Cohen, R., R. Daniel, et al. Onychotoxidermies. *Onychologie: Diagnostic, traitement, chirurgie.* R. K. Scher and C. R. Daniel III. French ed, Abimelec P, Elsevier 2007: p 193.

[22]   Horio T, Yokoyama M. Tegaful photosensitivity--lichenoid and eczematous types, *Photodermatol.* 1986;3:192-3.

[23]   Stevens HP, Ostlere LS, Begent RH, Dooley JS, Rustin MH, Pellagra secondary to 5-fluorouracil, *Br J Dermatol.* 1993;128:578-80.

[24]   Hague JS, Ilchyshyn A, Lichenoid photosensitive eruption due to capecitabine chemotherapy for metastatic breast cancer *Clin Exp Dermatol.* 2007;32:102-3.

[25]   Guillot B, Bessis D, Clinical appearance and management of cutaneous side effects of EGF receptor inhibitors A*nn Dermatol Venereol.* 2006 Dec;133(12):1017-20.

[26]   León-Mateos A, Zulaica A, Caeiro JL, Fabeiro JM, Calviño S, Peteiro C, Toribio, J.Photo-induced granulomatous eruption by hydroxyurea, *J Eur Acad Dermatol Venereol.* 2007;21:1428-9.

[27]   Yokote R, Tokura Y, Igarashi N, Ishikawa O, Miyachi Y, Photosensitive drug eruption induced by flutamide.*Eur J Dermatol. 1998 Sep;8:427-9.*

[28]   Mantoux F, Bahadoran P, Perrin C, Bermon C, Lacour JP, Ortonne JP. [Flutamide-induced late cutaneous], *Ann Dermatol Venereol.* 1999;126:150-2. French.

[29]   Hird AE, Wilson J, Symons S, Sinclair E, Davis M, Chow E, Radiation recall dermatitis: case report and review of the literature, *Curr Oncol.* 2008 Feb;15(1):53-62.

[30]   Camidge R, Price A. Characterizing the phenomenon of radiation recall dermatitis. *Radiother Oncol,* 2001;59:237–45.

[31]   Putnik K, Stadler P, Schafer C, Koelbl O. Enhanced radiation sensitivity and radiation recall dermatitis (rrd) after hypericin therapy—case report and review of the literature. *Radiat Oncol.* 2006;1:32.

[32]   Tan CT, Dargeon HW, Burchenal JH. The effect of actinomycin D on cancer in childhood. *Pediatrics.* 1959;24:544–61.

[33]   Sears ME. Erythema in areas of previous irradiation in patients treated with hydroxyurea (nsc-32065), *Cancer Chemother Rep.* 1964;40:31–2.

[34]   Nemechek PM, Corder MC. Radiation recall associated with vinblastine in a patient treated for Kaposi sarcoma related to acquired immune deficiency syndrome. *Cancer.* 1992;70:1605–6.

[35]   Solberg LA Jr, Wick MR, Bruckman JE. Doxorubicin-enhanced skin reaction after whole-body electron-beam irradiation for leukemia cutis. *Mayo Clin Proc.* 1980;55:711–15.

[36] Donaldson SS, Glick JM, Wilbur JR. Letter: Adriamycin activating a recall phenomenon after radiation therapy. *Ann Intern Med.* 1974;81:407–8.

[37] Heidary N, Naik H, Burgin S, Chemotherapeutic agents and the skin: An update.*J Am Acad Dermatol.* 2008;58:545-70.

[38] Wilson J, Carder P, Gooi J, Nishikawa H. Recall phenomenon following epirubicin, *Clin Oncol (R Coll Radiol), 1*999;11:424–5.

[39] Fontana JA. Radiation recall associated with vp-16–213 therapy. *Cancer Treat Rep.* 1979;63:224–5.

[40] Jaffe N, Paed D, Farber S, et al. Favorable response of metastatic osteogenic sarcoma to pulse high-dose methotrexate with citrovorum rescue and radiation therapy. *Cancer.* 1973;31:1367–73.

[41] Weiss RB, James WD, Major WB, Porter MB, Allegra CJ, Curt GA. Skin reactions induced by trimetrexate, an analog of methotrexate. *Invest New Drugs.* 1986;4:159–63.

[42] Perez EA, Campbell DL, Ryu JK. Radiation recall dermatitis induced by edatrexate in a patient with breast cancer, *Cancer Invest.* 1995;13:604–7.

[43] Parry BR. Radiation recall induced by tamoxifen. *Lancet.* 1992;340:49. 18.

[44] Raghavan VT, Bloomer WD, Merkel DE. Taxol and radiation recall dermatitis. *Lancet.* 1993;341:1354.

[45] Schweitzer VG, Julliard GJ, Bajada CL, Parker RG. Radiation recall dermatitis and pneumonitis in a patient treated with paclitaxel. *Cancer.* 1995;76:1069–72.

[46] Yeo W, Leung SF, Johnson PJ. Radiation-recall dermatitis with docetaxel: establishment of a requisite radiation threshold. *Eur J Cancer.* 1997;33:698–9.

[47] Stelzer KJ, Griffin TW, Koh WJ. Radiation recall skin toxicity with bleomycin in a patient with Kaposi sarcoma related to acquired immune deficiency syndrome, *Cancer.* 1993;71:1322–5. [.

[48] Castellano D, Hitt R, Cortes–Funes H, Romero A, Rodriguez– Peralto JL. Side effects of chemotherapy: case 2. Radiation recall induced by gemcitabine. *J Clin Oncol.* 2000;18:693–8.

[49] Chan RT, Au GK, Ho JW, Chu KW. Radiation recall with oxaliplatin: report of a case and review of the literature. *Clin Oncol (R Coll Radiol).* 2001;13:55–7.

[50] Kennedy RD, McAleer JJ. Radiation recall dermatitis in a patient treated with dacarbazine. *Clin Oncol (R Coll Radiol).* 2001;13:470–2.

[51] Ortmann E, Hohenberg G. Treatment side effects: case 1. Radiation recall phenomenon after administration of capecitabine. *J Clin Oncol.* 2002;20:3029–30.

[52] Thomas R, Stea B. Radiation recall dermatitis from high-dose interferon alfa-2b. *J Clin Oncol.* 2002;20:355–7.

[53] Ee HL, Yosipovitch G. Photo recall phenomenon: an adverse reaction to taxanes. *Dermatology.* 2003;207:196–8.

[54] Jimeno A, Cirelos EM, Castellano D, Caballero B, Rodriguez– Peralto JL, Cortes–Funes H. Radiation recall dermatitis induced by pegylated liposomal doxorubicin. *Anticancer Drugs.* 2003;14:575–6.

[55] Keung YK, Lyerly ES, Powell BL. Radiation recall phenomenon associated with arsenic trioxide. *Leukemia.* 2003;17:1417–36.

[56] Borgia F, Guarneri C, Guarneri F, Vaccaro M. Radiation recall dermatitis after docetaxel administration: absolute indication to replace the drug? *Br J Dermatol.* 2005;153:674–5.

[57]   Barlesi F, Tummino C, Taset AM, Astoul P. Unsuccessful rechallenge with pemetrexed after previous radiation recall dermatitis. *Lung Cancer.* 2006;54:423–5.

[58]   Saif MW, Black G, Johnson M, Russo S, Diasio R, Radiation recall phenomenon secondary to capecitabine: possible role of thymidine phosphorylase, *Cancer Chemother Pharmacol.* 2006; 58:771-5.

[59]   Jimeno A, Ciruelos EM, Castellano D, Caballero B, Rodriguez-Peralto JL,Cortés-Funes H., Radiation recall dermatitis induced by pegylated liposomal doxorubicin, *Anticancer Drugs,* 2003;14:575-6.

[60]   Amblard P, Photoprotection interne, *Photodermatologie,* Ed. Arnette 2008, p. 181.

[61]   Hoffmann K, Hanke D, Altmeyer P, UV-protective clothing in Europe. Recommandations of a European working party. *Eur J Dermatol,* 1997, 7: 240-241.

[62]   Gambichler T, Hatch KL, Avermaete has, Altmeyer P, Hoffmann K, Influence off wetness one the ultraviolet protection Factor (UPF) off textile: in vitro and in vivo measurements. *Photodermatol Photoimmunol Photomed.* 2002; 18: 29-35.

[63]   Green has, Williams G, Neale R, Hart V, Leslie D, Parsons P, Marks GC, Gaffney P, Battistutta D, Frost C, Lang C, Russell A. Daily sunscreen application and betacarotene supplementation in prevention off basal-concealment and squamous-concealment carcinomas of the skin: randomised controlled trial has. *Lancet.* 1999, 28; 354: 723-9.

[64]   Lee TK, Rivers JK, Gallagher RP. Site-specific protective effect of broad-spectrum sunscreen one nevus development among white schoolchildren in a randomized trial. *J Am Acad Dermatol.* 2005; 52: 786-92.

In: Handbook of Skin Care in Cancer Patients
Editors: Pierre Vereecken and Ahmad Awada

ISBN: 978-1-61668-419-8
© 2012 Nova Science Publishers, Inc.

Chapter 6

A CRITICAL REVIEW OF CUTANEOUS TOXICITY OF ANTICANCER TREATMENTS

Hans Prenen[1,2] and Ahmad Awada[2]

[1]Digestive Oncology Unit, UZ Gasthuisberg, Leuven, Belgium
[2]Department of Medical Oncology, Institute Bordet, Brussels, Belgium

ABSTRACT

Cutaneous reactions to chemotherapy are very common in clinical practice and may contribute significantly to the morbidity of cancer patients. Therefore, recognition and management of these side effects is important to provide optimal care. Chemotherapy-related cutaneous toxicity includes generalized rashes as well as site specific toxicity such as mucositis, nail changes or for example hand-foot syndrome. Most of these toxic effects are reversible with delay or dose reductions of chemotherapy. Newer anticancer targeted therapies may also be associated with cutaneous toxicity.

In this chapter we would like to give an overview of the most common cutaneous side effects of classical chemotherapy as well as the new monoclonal antibodies and tyrosine kinase inhibitors.

INTRODUCTION

Chemotherapy refers to the treatment of cancer by anti-neoplastic drugs. The first drug used for cancer treatment dates back to the early 20th century, which is mustard gas. Since then, many other drugs have been developed to treat cancer. The majority of chemotherapeutic drugs can be divided in to alkylating agents, antimetabolites, antracyclines, plant alkaloids and topoisomerase inhibitors. All of these drugs affect cell division or DNA synthesis in some way. The last decade, a significant number of new anticancer agents have been approved and used for the treatment of cancer, which have a totally different mechanism of action. These molecular-targeted drugs include monoclonal antibodies, tyrosine kinase inhibitors and anti-angiogenetic agents. Some of those agents give rise to specific mucocutaneous side effects.

This chapter reviews the most frequent cutaneous toxicity of as well the classic agents as the new molecular-targeted drugs. The presentation and severity of the skin toxicities depends on several factors such as dosing, type of agent and the functional status of the patient. A lot of different skin or nail toxicities have been reported and are overviewed in table 1. Although dermatologic complications are almost never fatal, they alter seriously the quality of life of the patients.

1. ALKYLATING AGENTS

Alkylating agents are cytotoxic drugs that place an alkyl group in place of a nucleophilic group in DNA, which inhibits DNA synthesis and therefore inhibits cancer cell growth (Table 2). Alkylating agents were among the first anti-cancer drugs and are the most commonly used agents in chemotherapy today. They are the major components of combination chemotherapy regimens.

Cyclophosphamide is used to treat various types of cancer and is a pro-drug that is converted in the liver to an active form. It is mainly used in combination with other chemotherapeutic agents. It may give rise to transverse bands or diffuse hyperpigmentation of the nails, teeth, mucosa, palms and soles [1]. Furthermore, urticaria,hypersensitivity and anaphylactic reactions have been reported [2]. Other alkylating agents that have been associated with hyperpigmentation are busulfan and ifosfamide. The mechanism of chemotherapy-induced hyperpigmentation reactions is currently unknown. In most cases, discoloration will gradually resolve after the discontinuation of the chemotherapy.

Alopecia is the most common dermatologic complication associated with chemotherapy. In the group of alkylating agents, alopecia is predominantly associated with busulfan, cyclophosphamide and ifosfamide treatment [3]. It is suggested that this toxicity is a result of the entry of lipophylic metabolites into the hair follicles [4].

Table 1a. Most common agents associated with skin or nail toxicity

Skin or nail Toxicity	Most common Agent		Skin or nail Toxicity	Most common Agent	
Maculo-papular rash	Cytarabine Cetuximab		Papulopu-stular rash	Cetuximab Erlotinib	Gefitinib Panitu-mumab
Hyper-pigmen-tation	5-FU Bleomycin Busulfan Cisplatin Cyclopho-sphamide Dactino-mycin Dauno-rubicin	Docetaxel Doxorubicin Ifosfamide Mitoxantrone Methotrexaat Procarbazine Vinorelbine	Neutro-phylic eccrine hydradenitis	Bleomycine Chlorambucil Cyclophosphamide Cytarabine Doxorubicine Lomustine Mitoxantrone	

Table 1a. (continued)

Skin or nail Toxicity	Most common Agent		Skin or nail Toxicity	Most common Agent	
Hyper-sensitivity reactions	Adriamycin Carboplatin Cisplatin Cladribine Cyclopho-sphamide Docetaxel	Etoposide Cetuximab Oxaliplatin Paclitaxel Panitumumab Rituximab	**Mucositis**	5-FU Antracyclines Cetuximab Cyclophospha mide Cytarabine	Dactinomycin Doceta-xel Methotrexate Paclitaxel Vinca-alkaloids
Alopecia	5-FU Bleomycin Cisplatin Cyclopho-sphamide Cytarabine Dacarba-zine Daunoru-bicin Dactino-mycin Docetaxal Doxorubicin	Etoposide Ifosfamide Irinotecan Mechlore-thamine Mitomycine C Paclitaxel Temozo-lomide Topotecan Vinblastine Vincristine	**Skin atrophy**	5-Fluoro-uracyl Hydroxyurea	
			Steven-Johnson syndrome Toxic epidermal necrolysis	5-Fluoro-uracyl Cytarabine Doxorubicin Gemcitabine Imatinib Methotrexaat	

Table 1b. Most common agents associated with skin or nail toxicity

Skin or nail Toxicity	Most common Agent		Skin or nail Toxicity	Most common Agent	
Inflam-mation of actinic keratosis	5-fluoro-uracil Cytarabine Doxorubicin	Sorafenib Sunitinib Vincristine	**Vascu-litis**	Gemcitabine Hydroxyurea	Methotrexate Pemetrexed
Hand-Foot syndrome	5-Fluoro-Uracil Bleomycine Capecitabine Cytarabine Docetaxel Doxorubicin Etoposide	Gemcitabine Hydroxyurea Methotrexate Peg-doxorubicin Sorafenib Sunitinib	**Radi-ation recall derma-titis**	5-FU Bleomycin Capecitabine Cyclopho-sphamide Cytarabine Daunorubicin Dactinomycin Docetaxel Doxorubicin	Etoposide Gemcitabine Hydroxyurea Lomustine Melphalan Methotrexate Paclitaxel Pemetrexed Vinblastine

Table 1b. (continued)

Skin or nail Toxicity	Most common Agent		Skin or nail Toxicity	Most common Agent	
Onycho-lysis	5-FU Bleomycine Capecitabine Cyclopho-sphamide	Docetaxel Doxorubicin Hydroxyurea Paclitaxel	Sclerosis	Bleomycin Docetaxel	Gemcitabine Paclitaxel
Ulcera-tion	Cisplatin Hydroxy-urea Methotrexate		Blistering derma-toses	Fludarabine Gemcitabine Paclitaxel	
Periun-gual inflame-mation	Cetuximab Docetaxel Etoposide	Gefitinib Paclitaxel Sunitinib Sorafenib	Splinter hemor-rhages	Imatinib Sorafenib Sunitinib	

Table 2. Alkylating agents

Alkylating agents

• Nitrogen Mustards
    Mechlorethamine (Nitrogen mustard)
    Melphalan
    Chlorambucil
    Cyclophosphamide
    Ifosfamide
    Busulfan
• Nitrosurea
    BCNU (Carmustine)
    Fotemustine
    Streptozocin
• Tetrazines
    Dacarbazine
    Temozolomide
• Aziridines
    Mitomycine C

2. PLATINUM AGENTS

The platinum agents are complexes of platinum with ligands that, like the alkylating agents, form strong chemical bonds in proteins and nucleic acids. They are non-specific cell cycle phase. The first platinum anti-tumour compound, discovered in the early 1970's is cisplatin. Cisplatin based chemotherapy is the cornerstone in the treatment of many cancers like testicular cancer, lymphoma, squamous cell carcinoma of the head and neck, ovarian cancer, bladder cancer, lung cancer, cervical cancer, oesophageal and stomach cancer.

The other members of this class include carboplatin and oxaliplatin which are less toxic than its parent compound cisplatin. Dose limiting side-effects include nausea and vomiting, myelosuppression, electrolyte disturbances, nephrotoxicity, neurotoxicity and ototoxicity. Minor alopecia is a possible dermatologic side effect. As another possible effect, with some implications at the cutaneous side cisplatin has been associated with severe vascular toxicity and arteritis [5]. This vascular phenomenon could lead in predisposed patients to cerebrovascular events and myocardial infarcts. Therefore, physicians should be aware of this possible complication in patients with cutaneous signs of arteritis.

Carboplatin, a second-generation platinum compound, is associated with less nephrotoxicity, neurotoxicity, ototoxicity and nausea than cisplatin. Hypersensitivity occurs in around 2% of patients and mainly seen after several cycles of carboplatin-based chemotherapy [6]. Interestingly, cisplatin has been safely administered without reaction, to some patients that developed an allergic reaction to carboplatin but this administration should be done under close surveillance [7].

Oxaliplatin is a third generation platinum compound that is mainly used for the treatment of metastatic colon and rectum carcinoma in combination with 5-Fluoro-Uracyl. After several course of therapy, oxaliplatin can cause a hypersensitivity reaction like carboplatin, including skin rash, pruritus, dyspnoea and anaphylaxis [8]. The rate is estimated to be between 2 and 12% [8].

There are case-reports in the literature of oxaliplatin-induced radiation recall [9].

3. ANTI-METABOLITES

Anti-metabolites are anti-neoplastic drugs with a similar structure to a metabolite required for normal biochemical reactions and therefore interfering with DNA production. Anti-metabolites are distinguished in three main groups which are the anti-folates, the purine and pyrimidine analogues (Table 3).

Table 3. Antimetabolites

Antifolates	Purine Analogues	Pyrimidine analogues
Methotrexate	Fludarabine	5-Fluoro-uracyl
Pemetrexed	Mercaptopurine	Capecitabine
Ralitrexed	Cladribine	Cytarabine (Ara C)
	Pentostatin	Gemcitabine
		Decitabine

Methotrexate (MTX), formerly known as amethopterin, is the anti-folate with the most extensive history and is used as a treatment in different types of cancer including acute lymphoblastic leukaemia. It acts by inhibiting the metabolism of folic acid. The most common adverse events are bone marrow suppression, nausea and vomiting, mucositis and renal toxicity.

Skin toxicity to MTX occurs in 5 to 10% of patients and manifests as an erythematous rash. It is rarely associated with acral erythema (hand-foot syndrome) but when causative, it may give rise to a bullous variant [10]. MTX has also been implicated in toxic epidermal necrolysis (TEN), also known as Lyell syndrome [11]. Methotrexate may also be phototoxic, leading to radiation recall from prior radiotherapy [12].

Pemetrexed (Alimta) is a new multitargeted antifolate that has demonstrated anti-tumour activity in mesothelioma and non-small cell lung cancer. The most commonly encountered toxicity is myelosuppression. Exanthema is the most commonly non-haematological side effect, present in 66% of patients in a phase II study [13]. Prophylactic dexamethasone can reduce the rate of rash to 17% in a subsequent phase III study [14]. Radiation recall dermatitis has been described in a few case-reports [15].

Fludarabine is a purine analogue, mainly used in hematological malignancies. Dermatologic adverse events are uncommon and include macular and papular rash and acral erythema [16]. Fludarabine has also been associated with paraneoplastic pemphigus (PNP) but it should be noted that it occurred in patients with CLL, which is a known factor associated with PNP [17].

Cladribine (2-CdA) is a chemotherapeutic drug, commonly used to treat lymphoproliferative disorders such as hairy cell leukaemia. In general this drug is very well tolerated. The most common adverse events are myelosuppression, fever, chills and fatigue. It has been associated with allergic cutaneous reactions and peripheral eosinophilia [18].

5-Fluoro-Uracyl (5-FU) is a pyrimidine analogue which principally acts as a thymidilate synthase inhibitor. It remains one of the most commonly used chemotherapeutics in the treatment of head and neck, breast, cervical and gastrointestinal cancer. The expression of 5-FU metabolic enzymes, such as thymidylate synthase, thymidine phosphorylase, orotate phosphoribosyl transferase and dihydropyrimidine dehydrogenase (DPD) has been examined in order to predict 5-FU sensitivity in several types of cancer. DPD is the initial enzyme in the catabolism of 5-FU, primarily in the liver. DPD is also the rate-limiting enzyme of 5-FU catabolism. 85% of the administered 5-FU is degraded to inactive metabolites by DPD. There are several situations, for example DPD deficiency, in which DPD activity is so decreased that severe and possible life-threatening 5-FU toxicity occurs. Capecitabine (Xeloda®) is an oral fluoropyrimidine prodrug that was designed to generate 5-FU preferentially in tumour tissue compared with healthy tissue. Capecitabine is metabolized to 5-FU via a three-step enzymatic process by subsequently carboxylesterase, cytidine deaminase and thymidine phosphorylase (TP). TP occurs at levels 3 to 10 times higher in tumor cells than in healthy tissue, which can enable selective drug activation of 5-FU at the tumor site and limit toxicity.

Dose-limiting toxicities of 5-FU are bone marrow suppression, nausea, vomiting, diarrhea and mucositis. Compared with 5-FU, capecitabine is associated with less stomatitis, alopecia, diarrhoea, nausea and neutropenia, but more hand-foot syndrome (HFS) [19].

The symptoms of HFS, also called palmar-plantar erythrodysesthesia, include numbness, paraesthesia, tingling, erythema, painless swelling and in more severe cases ulceration, desquamation or severe pain on the palms of the hands and/or the soles of the feet. The hands are usually more affected than the feet. The incidence of cumulative HFS observed with capecitabine is around 50% with 17% of patients reporting grade III toxicity [20]. Although it is not life-threatening, it affects quality of life and can lead to disruption of the treatment schedule and often leads to dosage reduction or treatment delay. HFS is dosage- and schedule dependent. Continuous infusion of 5-FU is associated with a higher incidence (up to 38%) of

HFS than bolus 5-FU administration (<5%). The causative mechanisms of HFS are still unknown. It is suggested that the presence of elevated TP expression in the palms of the hands along with an increased basal cell proliferation rate could be a causative mechanism for capecitabine-related HFS [21]. Interestingly, the addition of a DPD inhibitor significantly reduces the incidence of HFS, which suggests that the toxicity may be due to a by-product of DPD catabolism of the drug [22]. Evidence for this hypothesis comes from reports of DPD deficient patients that are at increased risk of severe toxicity from 5-FU, including grade IV myelosuppression and even death, where HFS is rarely reported as an adverse event [23]. Other dermatologic side-effects of 5-FU and capecitabine that are described in case reports are inflammation of actinic keratosis, cutaneous hyperpigmentation, radiation recall dermatitis, onycholysis and anoychmadesis (please check the exactitude of this word) [15].

Cytarabine, also known as Ara C, is an antimetabolic agent mainly used in the treatment of haematological malignancies such as leukaemia and non-hodgkin lymphoma. Main toxicities are bone marrow suppression, nausea, vomiting, mucositis, cerebellar toxicity and fever. Dermatologic side effects are rare but may occur with high-dose administration and are closely related to the duration of the treatment. Most frequent dermatological side effects are hand-foot syndrome [24], neutrophylic eccrine hydradenitis [25], morbiliform rashes [26], mucositis, alopecia and inflammation of actinic keratosis [27]. A less common side effect is leukocytoclastic vasculitis [28].

Gemcitabine is a nucleoside analogue used in various carcinomas as non-small cell lung cancer, pancreatic cancer, bladder cancer, ovarian cancer and breast cancer. In general it is very well tolerated. Dermatologic adverse events occur in about 30% of patients, the most common being alopecia (15%) and mild to moderate macular or papular rash (5-32%) [29]. It has also been reported to cause radiation recall dermatitis [30]. Other cutaneous side-effects described in case reports are bullous dermatitis, a pseudosclerodermatous reaction of the skin, hand-foot syndrome, vasculitis and steven-johnson syndrome [15]

4. ANTI-TUMOR ANTIBIOTICS

The anti-tumor antibiotics are antineoplastic agents derived from the streptomyces bacteria. They all inhibit either DNA synthesis or RNA transcription or both. The most important chemotherapeutic in this group include actinomycine-D, bleomycin, mitomycin and the antracyclines (doxorubicin, mitoxantrone, daunorubicin, idarubicin, epirubicin).

Dactinomycin (Actinomycine-D) was one of the first drugs to show significant antitumor effect in humans. The most common side effects include bone marrow suppression, nausea, vomiting, alopecia and mucositis [31]. Erythema characteristic of a radiation reaction in skin areas previously exposed to irradiation (radiation recall), is a well described phenomenon and can occur as long as 2 years after radiation [32]. Dactinomycin has also been associated with an erythematous linear pigmentation with follicular prominence and central desquamation [33].

Bleomycin is a cytostatic antibiotic discovered in 1965 and often used in poly-chemotherapeutic schemes for the treatment of testicular cancer, lymphomas and ovarian germ cell tumors. The most serious complication of bleomycin is pulmonary fibrosis and impaired lung function. Other side effects include fever.

The most commonly observed skin toxicities include alopecia, stomatitis and nail changes. Other less common side effects are the development of painful inflammatory nodules on the fingers, blisters, infiltrated violaceous plaques and hyperpigmentation [34]. A very unique pattern of hyperpigmentation induced by bleomycin is the so called "flagellate" hyperpigmentation, which mainly occurs on the thorax and back [35].

Anthracyclines are used to treat a wide variety of cancers including leukemias, lymphomas, lung, ovarian, uterine and breast cancer. They inhibit DNA and RNA synthesis by intercalating between base pairs of the DNA / RNA strand. Anthracyclines have also a topoisomerase II enzyme inhibitory effect. Anthracyclines are notorious for causing cardiotoxicity ranging from ECG changes to congestive heart failure. The cardiotoxicity is related to the patient's cumulative dose. Liposomal formulations of doxorubicin and daunorubicin have been developed to decrease the cardiotoxic effect.

Doxorubicin is together with daunorubicine the prototype of the anthracyclines and widely used in cancer chemotherapy. Acute side effects include nausea and vomiting, bone marrow toxicity and total alopecia. Some patients may develop hand-foot syndrome and severe skin reactions. Hand-foot syndrome is a common toxicity of the liposomal formulation of doxorubicin and it is mainly cumulative. An urticarial reaction, also known as the "adriamycin flare" has been reported in 3% of patients receiving doxorubicin [36]. Doxorubicin is also a radiosensitizer. Radiation recall has been reported in up to 43% of patients [37].

Idarubicin is an analogue of daunorubicin that is being used in the treatment of haematological malignancies. Cutaneous toxicities associated with idarubicin include alopecia, hand-foot syndrome, radiation recall dermatitis, stomatitis and pigmented bands of the nails [38-39].

5. PLANT DERIVATIVES (INCLUDING MICROTUBULE INHIBITORS AND PODOPHYLLOTOXIN COMPOUNDS)

Plant alkaloids are antimitotic agents, derived from plants that block cell division by preventing microtubule function. Microtubules are vital for cell division. The main examples are the vinca alkaloids, the taxanes and the podophyllotoxins.

The vinca alkaloids include vincristine, vinblastine, vinorelbine, vinflunine and vindesine. The dose-limiting toxicity of vincristin is neurotoxicity. The classic vinca alkaloids cause alopecia in 20 – 70% of patients. Vinorelbine has an improved safety profile over vincristine and vinblastine. Vinorelbine has been associated with hand-foot syndrome in four of sixty patients treated with high dose single agent vinorelbine for metastatic breast cancer [40]. This has not been observed with the lower dose schedules. Moderate to severe alopecia is noted in approximately 8% of vinorelbine-treated patients [41].

Taxanes are derived from the Pacific yew tree, Taxus brevifolia. They include paclitaxel and docetaxel and are one of the most powerful chemotherapeutic agents. Both drugs are frequently associated with cutaneous side effects, with an estimated incidence of 81%. Skin toxicities are more frequent with docetaxel than paclitaxel. Hand-foot syndrome has also been reported with docetaxel [42]. A variant of hand-foot syndrome called fixed erythrodysesthesia plaque (FEP) occurs as a fixed solitary erythematous plaque proximal to the infusion site after intravenous injection of docetaxel [43]. Other cutaneous toxicities reported with docetaxel include alopecia, mucositis, exanthemas, urticaria, radiation recall and nail changes including onycholysis [44]. Other nail changes include hyperpigmentation, splinter hemorrhage, subungual hyperkeratosis, orange discoloration and paronychia. The use of a frozen glove can significantly reduce the incidence of skin and nail toxicity associated with docetaxel [45]. Rarely, docetaxel has been associated with scleroderma-like changes [46].

Cutaneous toxicity of paclitaxel includes alopecia, hypersensitivity reactions, radiation recall dermatitis, erythema multiforme and onchylosis [15].

The epipodophyllotoxines teniposide and etoposide are semisynthetic derivatives of podophyllotoxin, a plant derived antimitotic agent. Etoposide causes alopecia in two-thirds of patients [47] and is rarely associated with hand-foot syndrome [48]. Etoposide has been reported to induce a morbilliform rash of erythematous macules and papules. This eruption begins about 1 week after start of the treatment and spontaneously resolves within 3 weeks [49].

6. Topoisomerase 1 Inhibitors

Topoisomerase inhibitors interfere with the topoisomerase enzymes, that control the changes in DNA structure. They have become popular targets for cancer treatment. The most familiar chemotherapeutics in this class are the topoisomerase I inhibitors irinotecan and topotecan. They act by breaking single-stranded DNA during replication. Topotecan is approved for the treatment of metastatic ovarian cancer, cervical cancer and small cell lung cancer. Common cutaneous toxicities include alopecia (77%) and maculopapular rash (6%) [50]. Topotecan has also been associated with a cellulite-like fixed drug eruption which decreases in severity with continuous therapy [51].

Irinotecan (CPT11) is a pro-drug, converted to the active metabolite SN-38 in the liver. Its main use is in colon cancer particularly in the regimen FOLFIRI (5-FU, Leucovorin, irinotecan) or in combination with cetuximab. The most significant side effects are severe diarrhea and myelosuppression. Alopecia occurs in 50% of patients [52].

7. Proteasome Inhibitors

Bortezomib is the first proteasome inhibitor approved for the treatment of multiple myeloma. The adverse events are usually mild, including diarrhea, nausea and vomiting, fatigue and peripheral neuropathy. An analysis of 140 patients with non-Hodgkin lymphomas who received bortezomib in monotherapy revealed 26 patients with an erythematous maculopapular or desquamative rash [53]. In general the cutaneous toxicity is mild.

8. Monoclonal Antibodies

Monoclonal antibodies are molecules that bind only to cancer-cell specific antigens and induce among other effects an immunological response against the target cancer cell. The most frequent used monoclonal antibodies in cancer medicine are trastuzumab, bevacizumab, rituximab, cetuximab and panitumumab.

Cetuximab and panitumumab are both monoclonal antibodies directed toward the extracellular ligand-binding domain of the Epidermal Growth-Factor Receptor (EGFR). The most commonly observed side effect with EGFR inhibitors is an acneiform eruption, which occurs in about 80% of patients [54]. The exact pathophysiology of this rash remains unclear and interestingly the skin toxicity seems to correlate to clinical outcome [55]. Other skin toxicities include nail fragility, hair changes and xerosis [56].

Trastuzumab is a humanized monoclonal antibody that acts on the HER2/Neu (erbB2) receptor and its principal use is as an anticancer agent in 20% breast cancer patients overexpressing the HER2/Neu receptor. The characteristic cutaneous side effects observed with EGFR-directed therapies have not been reported for therapies targeting HER2, such as trastuzumab. Infusion reactions consisting of hypotension, dyspnea and morbilliform rash are relatively frequent with monoclonal antibodies such as trastuzumab en rituximab [57].

Bevacizumab is the first anti-angiogenic agent, approved in combination with irinotecan and 5-FU based chemotherapy for the treatment of metastatic colorectal cancer. The most common adverse events of anti-angiogenic agents are hypertension, bleeding, trombosis, proteinuria and delayed wound healing. No specific skin toxicities have been reported.

9. TYROSINE KINASE INHIBITORS (TKI'S)

Tyrosine kinases play an important role in normal cellular regulatory processes. There are approximately 60 receptor tyrosine kinases that have been identified. Ligand binding induces dimerization of these receptors, resulting in autophosphorylation and activation of tyrosine kinase activity. Several small molecule inhibitors of tyrosine kinases have been developed and are already used in the clinic. The most common used inhibitors are summarized in Table 4.

The skin rash observed with EGFR inhibitors is more severe and diffuse with the monoclonal antibodies directed toward EGFR such as cetuximab (75 to 91%), than with small molecule tyrosine kinase inhibitors such as erlotinib (48 to 67%) and gefitinib (24 to 62%) [55, 58, 59]. Other skin toxicities such as nail fragility, hair changes and xerosis can also be present with TKI as observed with the antibodies against EGFR.

Imatinib is an oral drug that is approved for the treatment of chronic myeloid leukaemia and gastrointestinal stromal tumors. Most adverse events are mild including nausea, oedema, diarrhea and myalgia. Skin rash is also a common side effect observed in about 22% of patients treated with imatinib [60]. In most cases the rash manifests as erythematous macules and/or papules involving the whole body. Oedema manifests primarily periorbital. Severe cutaneous side-effects linked to imatinib are Steven-Johnson syndrome [61] and acute generalized exanthematous pustulosis [62]. Localized or generalized hypopigmentation is also commonly observed in 41% of patients treated with imatinib [63]. Possible cutaneous side-effects described in case reports include lichenoid eruptions, follicular mucinosis, a pityriasis rosea-like eruption, Sweet syndrome, neutrophylic eccrine hidradenitis, porphyria cutanea tarda and nail dystrophy [15].

Dasatinib is a multi-tyrosine kinase inhibitors and is associated with cutaneous side effects in about 35% of patients. These side effects include erythema, macular and popular eruptions and an exfoliative rash [64].

Sorafenib and sunitinib are both oral small-molecule multi-tyrosine kinase inhibitors, approved for the treatment of renal cell carcinoma. Most frequent cutaneous side effects observed with sorafenib are rash (66%), hand-foot syndrome (62%), alopecia (53%) and a dry skin (23%) [65]. Cutaneous toxicities in sunitinib treated patients include periorbital oedema (50%), dry skin, subungual splinter hemorrhages, stomatitis, hand-foot syndrome and transient yellow skin discoloration [66]. It is also frequent to observe reversible hair discoloration with sunitinib therapy.

Table 4. Tyrosine kinase inhibitors

Target	Inhibitor
Epidermal Growth Factor Receptor (EGFR)	Erlotinib
	Gefitinib
EGFR + HER2/Neu (ErbB-2)	Lapatinib
BCR-ABL, c-KIT, PDGFRα and β	Imatinib
	Nilotinib
Vascular Endothelial Growth Factor Receptor (VEGFR)	Valatinib (PTK787)
Multi-targeted inhibitors: VEGFR, PDGFR, KIT,Raf,…	Sunitinib
	Sorafenib

REFERENCES

[1] Shah PC, Rao KR, Patel AR. Cyclophosphamide-induced nail pigmentation. *Br J Dermatol* 1978;98:675-680.

[2] Thong BY, Leong KP, Thumboo J, Koh ET, Tang CY. Cyclophosphamide type I hypersensitivity in systemic lupus erythematosus. *Lupus* 2002;11:127-129.

[3] Gauci L, Serrou B. Changes in hair pigmentation associated with cancer chemotherapy *Cancer Treat Rep* 1980;64:193.

[4] Feil VJ, Lamoureux CH. Alopecia activity of cyclophosphamide metabolites and related compounds in sheep. *Cancer Res* 1974;34:2596-2598.

[5] İçli F, Karaoğuz H, Dinçol D, Demirkazik A, Günel N, Karaoğuz R, Uner A. Severe vascular toxicity associated with cisplatin-based chemotherapy. *Cancer* 1993;72:587-593.

[6] Meyer L, Zuberbier T, Worm M, Oettle H, Riess H. Hypersensitivity reactions to oxaliplatin: Cross-reactivity to carboplatin and the introduction of a desensitization schedule. *J Clin Oncol* 2002;20:1146-1147.

[7] Ottaiano A, Tambaro R, Greggi S, *et al.* Safety of cisplatin after severe hypersensitivity reactions to carboplatin in patients with recurrent ovarian carcinoma. *Anticancer Res* 2003;23:3465-3468.

[8] Garufi C, Cristaudo A, Vanni B, *et al.* Skin testing and hypersensitivity reactions to oxaliplatin. *Ann Oncol* 2003;14:497-498.

[9] Chan RT, Au GK, Ho JW, Chu KW. Radiation recall with oxaliplatin: Report of a case and a review of the literature. *Clin Oncol* (R Coll Radiol) 2001;13:55-57.

[10] Feizy V, Namazi MR, Barikbin B, Ehsani A. Methotrexate-induced acral erythema with bullous reaction. *Dermatol Online J* 2003;9:14.

[11] Harrison PV. Methotrexate-induced epidermal necrosis. *Br J Dermatol* 1987;116:867-869.

[12] Guzzo C, Kaidby K. Recurrent recall of sunburn by methotrexate. *Photodermatol Photoimmunol Photomed* 1995;11:55-56.

[13] Thödtmann R, Sauter T, Weinknecht S, *et al*. A phase II trial of pemetrexed in patients with metastatic renal cancer. *Invest New Drugs* 2003;21:353-358.

[14] Cohen MH, Johnson JR, Wang YC, Sridhara R, Pazdur R. FDA drug approval summary: Pemetrexed for injection (Alimta) for the treatment of non-small cell lung cancer. *Oncologist* 2005;10:363-368.

[15] Heidary N, Naik H, Burgin S. Chemotherapeutic agents and the skin: An update. *J Am Acad Dermatol* 2008;58:545-570.

[16] Nomdedeu J, Puig L, Martino R, Montagut M, Mateu R, Domingo-Albos A, Soler J, Moragas J. Peculiar acral erythematous eruption after fludarabine treatment. *Biol Clin Hematol* 1995;17:92-93.

[17] Gooptu C, Littlewood TJ, Frith P, *et al*. Paraneoplastic pemphigus: an association with fludarabine? *Br J Dermatol* 2001;144:1255-1261.

[18] Robak T, Blasinska-Morawiec M, Krykowski E, *et al*. 2-Chorodeoxyadenosine (cladribine)-related eosinophilia in patients with lymphoproliferative diseases. *Eur J Haematol* 1997;59:216-220.

[19] Cassidy J, Twelves C, Van Cutsem E, *et al*. First-line oral capecitabine therapy in metastatic colorectal cancer: a favorable safety profile compared with intravenous 5-fluorouracil/leucovorin. *Ann Oncol* 2002;13:566–575.

[20] Walko CM, Lindley C. Capecitabine: a review. Clin Ther 2005;27:23–44.

[21] Milano G, Etienne-Grimaldi MC, Mari M, *et al*.. Candidate mechanisms for capecitabine-related hand-foot syndrome. *Br J Clin Pharmacol 2008* March 13 (Epub ahead of print).

[22] Yen-Revollo JL, Goldberg RM, McLeod HL. Can inhibiting dihydropyrimidine dehydrogenase limit hand-foot syndrome caused by fluoropyrimidines? *Clin Cancer Res* 2008;14:8-13.

[23] Saif MW, Diasio R. Is capecitabine safe in patients with gastrointestinal cancer and dihydropyrimidine dehydrogenase deficiency? *Clin Colorectal Cancer* 2006;5:359–362.

[24] Baack BR, Burgdorf WHC. Chemotherapy-induced acral erythema. *J Am Acad Dermatol* 1991;24:457-461.

[25] Hurt MA, Halvorson RD, Petr FC Jr, Cooper JT Jr, Friedman DJ. Eccrine squamous syringometaplasia: a cutaneous sweat gland reaction in the histologic spectrum of 'chemotherapy-associated eccrine hidradenitis' and 'neutrophilic eccrine hidradenitis'. *Arch Dermatol* 1990;126:73-77.

[26] Herzig RH, Wolff SN, Lazarus HM, Phillips GL, Karanes C, Herzig GP. High-dose cytosine arabinoside therapy for refractory leukemia. *Blood* 1983;62:361-369.

[27] Kechijian P, Sadick NS, Mariglio J, Schulman P. Cytarabine-induced inflammation in the seborrheic keratoses of Leser-Trélat. *Ann Intern Med* 1979;91:868-869.

[28] Ahmed I, Chen KR, Nakayama H, Gibson LE. Cytosine arabinoside-induced vasculitis. *Mayo Clin Proc* 1998;73:239-242.

[29] Chu CY, Yang CH, Chiu HC. Gemcitabine-induced acute lipodermatosclerosis-like reaction. *Acta Derm Venereol* 2001;81:426-428.

[30] Schwarts BM, Khuntia D, Kennedy AW, Markman M. Gemcitabine-induced radiation recall dermatitis following whole pelvic radiation therapy. *Gynecol Oncol* 2003;91:421-422.

[31] Benjamin RS, Hall SW, Burgess MA, *et al.* A pharmacokinetically based phase I-II study of single-dose actinomycin D (NSC-3053). *Cancer Treat Rep* 1976;60:289-291.

[32] Coppes MJ, Jorgenson K, Arlette JP. Cutaneous toxicity following the administration of dactinomycin. *Med Pediatr Oncol* 1997;29:226-227.

[33] Wyatt AJ, Leonard GD, Sachs DL. Cutaneous reactions to chemotherapy and their management. *Am J Clin Dermatol* 2006;7:45-63.

[34] Bronner AK, Hood AF. Cutaneous complications of chemotherapeutic agents. *J Am Acad Dermatol* 1983;9:645-663.

[35] Vuerstaek JD, Frank J, Poblete-Gutiérrez P. Bleomycin-induced flagellate dermatitis. *Int J Dermatol* 2007;46:3-5.

[36] Vogelzang NJ. "Adriamycin flare": a skin reaction resembling extravasation. *Cancer Treat Rep* 1979;63:2067-2069.

[37] Arthur DW, Koo D, Zwicker RD, *et al.* Partial breast brachytherapy after lumpectomy: low-dose-rate and high-dose-rate experience. *Int J Radiat Oncol Biol Phys* 2003;56:681-689.

[38] Gabel C, Eifel PJ, Tornos C, Burke TW. Radiation recall reaction to idarubicin resulting in vaginal necrosis. *Gynecol Oncol* 1995;57:266-269.

[39] Borecky DJ, Stephenson JJ, Keeling JH, Vukelja SJ. Idarubicin-induced pigmentary changes of the nails. *Cutis* 1997;59:203-204.

[40] Hoff PM, Valero V, Ibrahim N, Willey J, Hortobagyi GN. Hand-foot syndrome following prolonged infusion of high doses of vinorelbine. *Cancer* 1998;82:965-969.

[41] Fumoleau P, Delgado FM, Delozier T, *et al.* Phase II trial of weekly intravenous vinorelbine in first-line advanced breast cancer chemotherapy. *J Clin Oncol* 1993;11:1245-1152.

[42] Zimmerman GC, Keeling JH, Burris HA, *et al.* Acute cutaneous reactions to docetaxel, a new chemotherapeutic agent. *Arch Dermatol* 1995;131:202-206.

[43] Chu CY, Yang CH, Yang CY, Hsiao GH, Chiu HC. Fixed erythrodysaesthesia plaque due to intravenous injection of docetaxel. *Br J Dermatol* 2000;142:808-811.

[44] Susser WS, Whitaker-Worth DL, Grant-Kels JM. Mucocutaneous reactions to chemotherapy. *J Am Acad Dermatol* 1999;40:367-398.

[45] Scotté F, Tourani JM, Banu E, *et al.* Multicenter study of a frozen glove to prevent docetaxel-induced onycholysis and cutaneous toxicity of the hand. *J Clin oncol* 2005;23:4424-4429.

[46] Extra JM, Rousseau F, Bruno R, Clavel M, Le Bail N, Marty M. Phase I and pharmacokinetic study of taxotere (RP 56976;NSC 628503) given as a short intravenous infusion . *Cancer Res* 1993;53:1037-1042.

[47] Fontana JA. Radiation recall associated with VP-16-213 therapy. *Cancer Treat Rep* 1979;63:224-225.

[48] Portal I, Cardenal F, Garcia-del-Muro X. Etoposide-related acral erythema. *Cancer Chemother Pharmacol* 1994;34:181.

[49] Yokel BK, Friedman KJ, Farmer ER, Hood AF. Cutaneous pathology following etoposide therapy. *J Cutan Pathol* 1987;14:326-330.

[50] Creemers GJ, Wanders J, Gamucci T, *et al.* Topotecan in colorectal cancer: a phase II study of the EORTC early clinical trials group. *Ann Oncol* 1995;6:844-846.

[51] Senturk N, Yanik F, Yildiz L, Aydin F, Canturk T, Turanli AY. Topotecan-induced cellulitis-like fixed drug eruption. *J Eur Acad Dermatol Venereol* 2002;16:414-416.

[52] Rothenberg ML, Cox JV, DeVore RF, *et al.* A multicenter phase II trial of weekly irinotecan (CPT-11) in patients with previously treated colorectal carcinoma. *Cancer* 1999;85:786-795.

[53] Gerecitano J, Goy A, Wright J, *et al.* Drug-induced cutaneous vasculitis in patients with non-Hodgkin lymphoma treated with the novel proteasome inhibitor bortezomib: A possible surrogate marker of response? *Br J Haematol* 2006;134:391-398.

[54] Cunningham D, Humlet Y, Siena S, *et al.* Cetuximab monotherapy and cetuximab plus irinotecan in irinotecan-refractory metastastic colorectal cancer. *N Engl J Med* 2004;351:337-345.

[55] Perez-Soler R. Can rash associated with HER1/EGFR inhibition be used as a marker of treatment outcome? *Oncology* (Williston Park) 2003;17:23-28.

[56] Widakowich C, de Castro G, de Azambuja E, Dinh P, Awada A. Review: side effects of approved molecular targeted therapies in solid cancer. *Oncologist* 2007;12:1443-1455.

[57] Dillman RO. Infusion reactions associated with the therapeutic use of monoclonal antibodies in the treatment of malignancy. *Cancer Metast Rev* 18:465-471.

[58] Cohen EE, Rosen F, Stadler WM, *et al.* Phase II trial of ZD1839 in recurrent or metastatic squamous cell carcinoma of the head and neck. *J Clin Oncol* 2003;21:1980-1987.

[59] Kris MG, Natale RB, Herbst RS, *et al.* Efficacy of gefinitib, an inhibitor of the epidermal growth factor receptor tyrosine kinase, in symptomatic patients with non-small cell lung cancer: A randomized trial. *JAMA* 2003;290:2149-2158.

[60] Talpaz M, Silver RT, Druker BJ, *et al.* Imatinib induces durable hematologic and cytogenetic responses in patients with accelerated phase chronic myeloid leukaemia: Results of a phase 2 study. *Blood* 2002;99:1928-1937.

[61] Sanchez-Gonzales B, Pascual-Ramirez JC, Fernandez-Abellan P, Belinchon-Romero I, Rivas C, Vegara-Aguilera G. Severe skin reaction to imatinib in a case of Philadelphia-positive acute lymphoblastic leukaemia. *Blood* 2003;101:2446.

[62] Schwarz M, Kreuzer KA, Baskaynak G, Dorken B, le Coutre P. Imatinib-induced acute generalized exanthematous pustulosis (AGEP) in two patients with chronic myeloid leukaemia. *Eur J Haematol* 2002;69:254-256.

[63] Arora B, Kumar L, Sharma A, Wadhwa J, Kochupillai V. Pigmentary changes in chronic myeloid leukaemia patients treated with imatinib mesylate. *Ann Oncol* 2004;15:358-359.

[64] Talpaz M, Shah NP, Kantarjian H, *et al.* Dasatinib in imatinib-resistant Philadelphia chromosome-positive leukemias. *N Engl J Med* 2006;354;2531-2541.

[65] Ratain MJ, Eisen T, Stadler WM, *et al.* Phase II placebo-controlled randomized discontinuation trial of sorafenib in patients with metastatic renal cell carcinoma. *J Clin Oncol* 2006;24:2505-2512.

[66] Faivre S, delbaldo C, Vera K, *et al*. Safety, pharmacokinetic, and antitumor activity of SU11248, a novel oral multitarget tyrosine kinase inhibitor, in patients with cancer. *J Clin Oncol* 2006;24:25-35.

In: Handbook of Skin Care in Cancer Patients   ISBN: 978-1-61668-419-8
Editors: Pierre Vereecken and Ahmad Awada   © 2012 Nova Science Publishers, Inc.

Chapter 7

PRESSURE ULCERS OF CANCER PATIENTS

Patricia Senet[1], and Olivier Chosidow[2]

[1]Department of Dermatology, Assistance Publique Hôpitaux de Paris, Hôpital Tenon,
75020 Paris, France
[2]Department of Dermatology, Assistance Publique Hôpitaux de Paris, Hôpital Henri
Mondor, 94010 Créteil Cedex, France

ABSTRACT

Pressure ulcers are ischemic tissue damages, localised to the skin and the underlying tissues. They are mainly caused by extrinsic factors such as interface pressure, in patients presenting autonomy impairment. Pressure ulcer prevalence varies greatly by clinical setting but remains high, up to 10,5% in hospitals. The Norton Scale and the Braden Scale are the principal prediction tools for evaluating individual patient risk for pressure ulcer development, when used as an adjunct to the clinical judgement. Prevention and treatment are based on skin and local wound care, repositionning, use of pressure relieving support surfaces, nutritional support and surgery in some cases and for selcted localizations as trochanteric area. Pressure ulcers are associated with an increase in mortality rates, and health costs. Thus, prevention is critical to reduce their prevalence in hospital settings and long term care.

INTRODUCTION

A pressure ulcer is defined as an area of ischemic localised damage to the skin and underlying tissue resulting from compression between a bony prominence and an external surface. Pressure ulcers are mainly caused by pressure but also by shear, friction, or a combination of these factors [1,2]. The development of pressure ulcers may interfere with functionnal recovery, be complicated by pain and infection, contribute to increase of hospital length of stay and, to premature mortality in some patients [3,4]. Studies estimated that the cost of treatment per patient ranged between $500 and 100 000, depending on the location [5]. Prevention is usually considered as the most efficient and the less costly method to tackle the problem. Therefore, since 15 years, several quidelines have been published by national health authorities or international panel of experts to help preventing and treating pressure ulcers [1,2,6,7]. The epidemiology of pressure ulcers varies considerably by clinical setting and because of differences in performance of each survey. Incidence rates range from 0.4% to 38% in acute care, 2.2 to 23.9% in long-term care, 0 to 17% in home care [5,8]. A recent study have measured the pressure ulcer prevalence in 25 hospitals in 5 European countries. The pressure ulcer prevalence was 18.1% and 10.5%. when grade 1 ulcers were excluded. The sacrum and the heels were the most affected locations and only 9.7% of the patients received fully adequate preventive care [9].

Cancer, as pressure ulcers, is predminantly a disease of older adults. Moreover, cancer patients are at high risk of impairment of autonomy and a large proportion of them had rehabilitation needs on admission [10], indicating a high risk of pressure ulcer development.

PATHOGENESIS AND RISK ASSESSMENT

Risk factors of pressure ulcers are usually defined as extrinsic and intrinsic factors [1,11]. Extrinsic factors are interface pressure, shear, friction and moisture [2]. Ulceration develops when the pressure is sufficient (> 32 mmHg), to occlude the capillary skin bed, restricting blood flow and reducing lymphatic drainage, leading to tissue necrosis. Concurrent shearing forces damage the arterioles, interrupting the microcirculation, and activating clotting system. Frictional forces and excessively moist environment may lead to the formation of superficial skin erosions and increase the deleterious effects of pressure and friction [12,13]. Intrinsic factors are mainly a previous history of pressure damage, acute illness, increased age, immobility, low level of consciousness or sedation, sensory impairment, malnutrition, severe chronic or terminal disease, vascular disease, deshydratation and hypotension [6,12,14], old age and immobikity being probably the major risk factors.

The Norton Scale and the Braden Scale are the most widely used validated prediction tools for evaluating the individual patient risk for pressure ulcer development. The Norton Scale (table 1) is composed of 5 broad clinical categories: physical condition, mental state, activity, mobility and incontinence, a score of 16 or less indicating increased risk for pressure ulcer development. The Braden Scale (table 2) is composed of 6 broad clinical categories: sensory perception, moisture, activity, mobility, nutrition, friction and shear, a score of 18 or less indicating increased risk for pressure ulcer development. Although risk assessment scales predict the occurrence of pressure ulcers to some extent, there is no evidence that the routine use of these scales decreases pressure ulcer incidence [3,15], probably because it doesn't lead to efficient use of preventive measures [16, 17]. The Braden Scale offers the best balance between sensitivity and specificity and the best risk estimate. Both the Braden and Norton Scales are more accurate than nurses' clinical judgement in predicting pressure ulcer risk [8,16]. The risk assessment scales should be used as an adjunct to, not a substitute for, clinical judgement [1,2,6].

Table 1. Norton scale: Scores of 16 or less rate the patient «at risk»

A **Physical condition**	B **Mental condition**	C Activity	D Mobility	E Incontinence
Good **4**	Alert **4**	Ambulant **4**	Full **4**	Not **4**
Fair **3**	Apathic **3**	Walk/help **3**	Slightly **3**	Occasional **3**
Poor **2**	Confused **2**	Chairbound **2**	Limited **2**	Usually-urine **2**
Very bad **1**	Stupor **1**	Bedridden **1**	Very limited, immobile **1**	Doubly **1**
Total A	Total B	Total C	Total D	Total E

Table 2. Braden scale

Sensory perception (ability to respond meaningfully to pressure-related discomfort)	Completely limited 1	Very limited 2	Slightly limited 3	No impairment 4
Moisture (degree which skin is exposed to moisture)	Constantly moist 1	Very moist 2	Occasionally moist 3	Rarely moist 4
Activity (degree of physical activity)	bedfast 1	Chairfast 2	Walks occasionally 3	Walks frequently 4
Nutrition (usual food intake)	Very poor 1	Probably inadequate 2	Adequate 3	Excellent 4
Friction and shear	Problem 1	Potential problem 2	No apparent problem 3	

The lower the score the greater the risk of pressure ulcer. Usually a cut-off score of 18 is used to classify a patient «at risk» or «not at risk».

Table 3. European Pressure Ulcer Advisory Panel's classification of pressure ulcers

Grade 1	Non-blanchable erythema of intact skin. Discoloration, warmth, induration, or hardness of skin may also be used as indicators particularly in people with darker skin.
Grade 2	Partial-thickness skin loss, involving epidermis, dermis or both. This ulcer is superficial and presents clinically as an abrasion or blister
Grade 3	Full-thickness skin loss involving damage to or necrosis of subcutaneous tissue that may extend down to, but not though, underlying fascia.
Grade 4	Extensive destruction, tissue necrosis or damage to muscle, bone, or supporting structures, with or without full-thickness skin loss.

CLASSIFICATION

Various classification schemes are actually available but the European Pressure Ulcer Advisory Panel classification (Table 3, fig 1), in 4 grades, is actually the most used and recommended [2].

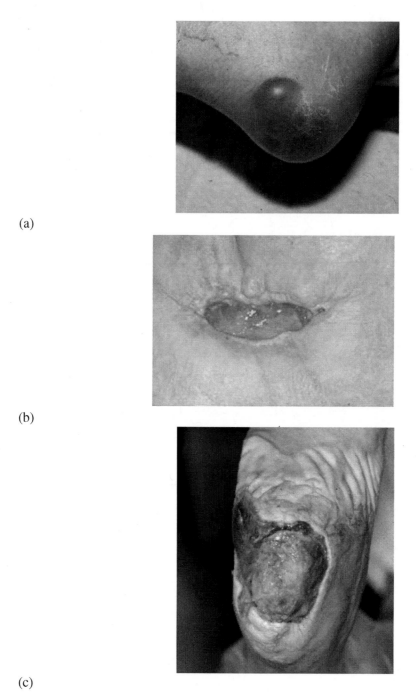

(a)

(b)

(c)

Figure 1. Grade of pressure ulcers. (a) Grade 2; (b) Grade 3; (c) Grade 4.

PREVENTION AND TREATMENT

1. Skin Care

Inspection of the skin should be performed at least once daily, specially on bony prominences to detect non-blanchable erythema of intact skin that is already a grade 1 pressure ulcer. Specific lotions or fatty acid preparations are often used by the care givers but no topical product has been correctly evaluated in prevention of pressure ulcers. Skin over bony prominences should be only inspected and cleaned, but not be massaged or rubbed, as this will exacerbate friction and could cause tissue damage [18]. Increase in moisture and humidity from urinary or fecal incontinence or perspiration may exacerbate skin maceration and is prevented by the use of absorbent underpads.

2. Assessment of Pressure Ulcer and Local Wound Care

The evaluation of a pressure ulcer, at least once weekly, should take into account the wound stage (deepth) and its characteristics such as amount of exudate, presence of necrotic tissue, granulation tissue, epithelialization, tunneling etc. Several tools have been develop to assess the healing of pressure ulcers. The most widely used is the PUSH (Pressure Ulcer Scale for Healing) that is composed of 3 wound characteristics: size of the wound (length and width), exudate amount and tissus type [19]. Irrigation with normal saline can be used for cleaning the ulcers as many antiseptics have shown to be cytotoxic, may induce contact dermatitis and may in fact delay granulation and epthelialization [20]. Topical antibiotics are not recommended for local wound care of chronic wounds, and if they were used, it should be limited for short periods only. In fact, topical antibiotics do not seem superior to normal saline for the prevention of bacterial growth [21] and contact dermatitis, systemic absorption, and moreover, development of bacterial resistance may occur with their prolongated used [22].

Since the 60's, it is has been recognized that optimal wound healing can be achieved when the wound is kept in a moist environment leading to the development of occlusive or semi-occlusive modern dressings. The choice of the ideal dressing according to the type of wound remains controversial. Clinical practice guidelines published on pressure ulcers, leg ulcers or diabetic foot ulcers, and systematic reviews on the treatment of arterial leg ulcers or surgical wounds, don't give enough indication to determine the strategy of local care for each type of wounds. However, there is a good evidence to suggest that hydrocolloid dressings are more efficient in term of complete healing than saline gauze or paraffin gauze for the treatment of chronic wounds. As alginates, used in single treatment or in a sequential strategy, are more efficient in term of wound area reduction than other modern dressings in treatment of chronic wounds, they may faster the debridment stage. Hydrocolloids and foam dressings seem to be equally efficient for optimizing the complete healing rate of chronic wounds [23].

3. Repositionning

Most guidelines recommend to turn the beddridden patients every 2 hours at least, to reduce interface pressure [12], although the ideal frequency of the patient repositionning has been poorly evaluated [3]. In fact, the frequency needed for repositionning is dependant of the level of pressure ulcer risk and of the pressure relief support surface that is used. Positionning patient on the femoral trochanter should be avoided. The patient is rather turned alternatively from the back to the right side and from the back to the left side. The position on the side is stabilized by cushions, with an angle of 30° between the bed and the pelvis. Lifting devices are used for patient repositionning to avoid friction and shear induced by dragging the patient during transfer, and the pressure is minimised on the ischial tuberosities and on the heels when the head of the bed is maintained at less than 30°. In wheelchairs, patients should performed position shifts at least every 30 minutes when possible and be sitted on pressure relieving cushion (air, gel or foam cushion).

4. Pressure Relieving Support Surfaces

Specialized support surfaces (matresses, beds and cushions) reduce the interface pressure between the patient and the support. Patients at high risk of pressure sore development, including bedridden patients and patients with pressure ulcers, should not be placed on ordinary foam mattresses and should have access to appropriate relieving support surfaces [6,24]. Pressure reducing surfaces may be either static support surfaces such as mattresses or mattress overlays, filled with air, water, gel, foam or a combination of these. Dynamic support surfaces include alternating-pressure matresses or mattress overlays (producing alternating low pressures between the patient and the surface), low-air-loss beds or mattresses where warmed air continually passed, including or not sensors for automatic monitoring of interface pressures, and air-fluidized matresses (silicone-coated beads and air) [13]. The relative merits of the different support surfaces are still unclear [24], however professional consensus [1,6] recommends that:

- in prevention, for patient with low- to-moderate risk of pressure sores, (no pressure sore, able to move himself in the bed and beddriden less than 15 hours/day), static supports are indicated (overlays or matresses)
- in prevention for patients at high risk of pressures sores (patient without any pressure sore and no able to move himself in the bed and beddriden more than 15 hours/day), or in treatment for patient with pressure sore grade 1 to 2, static supports are at least indicated, and alternating-pressure matresses or mattress overlays are recommended
- in treatment of grade 3 to 4 pressure sores, or in case of deterioration of affected areas or if further pressure ulcer develops, alternating-pressure matresses or mattress overlays are at least indicated, and low-air-loss beds or mattresses, or air fluidised are recommended.

5. Nutrition

A recent systematic review and meta-analysis shows that enteral nutritional support and, in particular high protein nutritional supplements, is associated with a significant reduction (by 25%) in pressure ulcer development. Oral nutrional support and enteral tube feeding may also aid pressure ulcer healing in at-risk patients groups but these trends require confirmation [25]. Nevertheless, , there is a consensus that nutrition is an important factor in both prevention and treatment of pressure ulcers [6]. Nutritional assessment include the mesure of height and weight (combined as body mass index), presence or not of undesired weight loss greater than 10% of normal body weight in the past 6 months, nutritional intake over the past 1, 3 or 7 days, and biochemical measurements such as serum albumin, haemoglobin and C reactive protein [26]. The primary goal of nutritional intervention is to correct protein-energy malnutrition, ideally though oral feeding. If both normal feeding nd protein-rich oral supplements fail to resolve malnutrition, then tube feeding may be undertaken, although risks sould be considered. General guidance is that individual may require a minimum of 30-35 kcal per kg body weight per day, with 1-1.5 g/kg/day protein required. When patients have established pressure ulcers, a similar strategy of nutritional intervention should be considered, although the demands may be greater [26]. Protein and calorie supplementation, with the use of arginine, vitamins and trace elements appear to have a positive effect on healing but the evidence for the value of other nutriments (vitamin C, zinc, etc) is weak [5,25,26]. Oversupplementing patients who do not have protein, vitamins or mineral deficiencies should be avoided [5,6].

6. Surgery

Surgery is usually considered once extrinsic and intrinsic factors have been resolved, in patients with grade 3 or 4 ulcers. Surgical management of pressure ulcers can be subdivided into 3 subtypes that may be combined: drainage or abscess surgery, debridment (superficial or with bone tissue removal), and closure sugery using direct closure, skin grafting or flap closure. Despite the lack of evidence that surgery is effective in the treatment of pressure ulcers and which techniques are the most effective, surgery is clearly indicated as a treatment option [6]. Recurrence rates are high and may reach 50% [18]. Identifying candidates to surgery may be based on overall assessment of the individual, taking specially into account nutritional status, aneasthesic risk, recurrence risk and ulcer location. Ischial and trochanteric areas are good indications for surgery, rather than heel and sacral areas.

INFECTIONS

Distinction between bacterial colonization and bacterial infection is important. Colonization can be defined as the presence of replicating microorganisms adherent to the wound in the absence of tissue damage. Wound infection can be defined as the presence of replicating organisms within a wound with subsequent host injury [27]. Clinical sign of wound infection include increased pain and exudate, erythema, oedema, abnormal smell, discoloration and delayed healing [28]. The recognition of bacterial colonization as a normal process seen in open wounds makes the interpretation of bacteriological culture results difficult. Wound swab cultures taken from pressure ulcers reveal polymicrobial growth, including aerobic organisms, such as Staphylococcus aureus or Streptococcus group A, Pseudomonas Aeruginosa, Enterobacter spp., and anaerobic organisms. Swab cultures may not reflect deep tissue cultures [27]. Bacterial load greater than 100 000 organisms or colony forming units per gram of tissue or mm^3 of pus is a predictor of wound infection [29,30] but biopsy of the ulcer with quantitative cultures of the tissue is rarely performed in routine practice. Bacterial cultures to confirm the organism and the antibiotic sensivities are more often obtained by aspiration, collection of pus or by sharp debridment with a scalpel. Antibiotics are often started empirically, covering Staphylococcus aureus, Streptococcus group-A and gram-negative rods.

Secondary bacteriema, septicaemia osteomyelitis and fistulas may complicate pressure ulcers, requiring adapted antibiotics and surgical drainage.

REFERENCES

[1]   www.has-sante.fr/portail/jcms/c_271996
[2]   www.epuap.org/grading.html
[3]   Reddy M, Gill SS, Rochon PA. Preventing pressure ulcers: a systematic review. *JAMA* 2006 ;296:974-84.
[4]   Thomas DR, Goode PS, Tarquine PH, Allman AM. Hospital-acquired pressure ulcers and risk of death. *J Am Geriatr Soc* 1996 ;44:1435-40.
[5]   Lyder CH. Pressure ulcer prevention and management. *JAMA* 2003 ;289:223-26.
[6]   www.nice.org.uk/CG029
[7]   Agency for Healthcare Research and Quality. www.ahrq.gov/clinic.
[8]   Bergstrom N, Braden B, Kemp M et al. Multi-site study of incidence of pressure ulcers and the relationship between risk level, demographic characteristics, diagnoses and prescription of preventive intervntions. *J Am Geriatr Soc* 1996 ;44:22-30.
[9]   Vanderwee K, Clak M, Dealey C et al. Pressure ulcer prevalence in Europe: a pilot study. *J Eval Clin Pract* 2007 ;13:227-35.
[10] Movsas SB, Chang VT, Tunkel RS et al. Rehabilitation needs of an inpatient medical oncology unit. *Arch Phys Med Rehabil* 2003 ;1642-46.
[11] Baumgarten M, Margolis D, Berlin JA et al. Risk factors for pressure ulcers among elderly hip fracture patients. *Wound Rep Reg* 2003 ;11: 96-103.
[12] Grey JE, Enoch S, Harding KG. ABC of wound healing. Pressure ulcers. *Br Med J* 2006 ;332: 472-75.
[13] Jones J. Evaluation of pressure ulcer prevention devices: a critical review of the literature. *J Wound Care* 2005 ;14: 422-425.
[14] De Laat EHEW, Schoonhoven L, Picckers P et al. Epidemiology, risk and prevention of pressure ulcers in critically ill patients: a literature review. *J Wound Care* 2006 ;15: 269-75.
[15] Schoonhoven L, Haalboom JRE, Algra A et al. Prospective cohort study of routine use of risk assessment scales for prediction of pressure ulcers. *Br Med J* 2002 ;325: 797.

[16] Pancorbo-Hidalgo PL, Garcia-Fernandez FP, lopez-medina IM, Alvarez-Nieto C. Risk assessment scales for pressure ulcer prevention: a systematic review. *J Adv Nurs* 2006 ; 54: 94-110.

[17] Brown SJ. The braden Scale. *Orthopaedic Nursing* 2004 ;23: 30-8.

[18] Kanj LF, Wilking SVB, Phillips TJ. Pressure ulcers. *J Am Acad Dermatol* 1998 ;38: 517-36.

[19] Stotts NA, Rodehaver GT, Thoma DR et al. An instrument to measure healing in pressure ulcers: development and validation of the Pressure Ulcer Scale for Healing (PUSH) *J Gerontol* 2001 ;56: M795-M799.

[20] Wolkenstein P., Vaillant L. Les antiseptiques en peau lésée. *Ann Dermatol Venerol* 1996 ; 123: 343-348.

[21] White RJ, Cutting K, Kingsley A. Topical antimicrobials in the control of wound bioburden. *Ostomy Wound Manage* 2006 ;52: 26-58.

[22] Machet L, Wolkenstein P, Vaillant L. Topical antibiotics used in dermatology: efficiency, indications and adverse effects. *Ann Dermatol Venereol* 2000 ;127: 425-31.

[23] Chaby G, Senet P,Vaneau M, Martel P, Guillaume JC, Meaume S, Téot L et coll. Dressings for acute and chronic wounds: a systematic review. *Arch Dermatol* 2007 ;143: 1297-304.

[24] Cullum N, Mc Innes E, Bell-Syer SEM, Legood R. Support surfaces for pressure ulcer prevention. Cochrane Database of Systematic reviews 2004, *Issue 3.* Art.N°: CD001735.

[25] Stratton RJ, Ek AC, Engfer M et al. Enteral nutritional support in prevention and treatment of pressure ulcers: A systematic review and meta-analysis. *Ageing Res Rev* 2005 ;4: 422-50.

[26] Clark M, Schols JMGA, Benati G et al. Pressure ulcers and nutrition: a new European Guideline. *J Wound care* 2004 ;13: 267-72.

[27] Edwards R, Harding KG. Bacteria and wound healing. *Curr Opin Infect Dis* 2004 ;17: 91-6.

[28] Cutting KF, White RJ. Criteria for identifying wound infection-revisited. *Ostomy/Wound Manage* 2005 ;51: 28-34.

[29] Bowler PG. The 105 bacterial growth guideline: reassessing its clinical relevance in wound healing. *Ostomy/Wound Manage* 2003 ;49: 44-53.

[30] Healy B, Freedman A. ABC of wound healing. Infections. *Br Med J* 2006 ;332: 838-841.

In: Handbook of Skin Care in Cancer Patients
Editors: Pierre Vereecken and Ahmad Awada

ISBN: 978-1-61668-419-8
© 2012 Nova Science Publishers, Inc.

Chapter 8

HOW DERMATOPATHOLOGY CAN BE USEFUL IN THE COMPREHENSION OF THERAPEUTIC AND SIDE EFFECTS OF NOVEL BIOLOGICALLY TARGETED THERAPIES

Laporte Marianne

Dermatopathology, Free University of Brussels, Belgium

ABSTRACT

Dermatology and dermatopathology could provide some useful tools in the management of anti-EGFR treatments from two points of view:

-clinical symptoms such as rash can be the signal of effectiveness of treatments by cetuximab,ABX-EGF and erlonitib.

-immunochemistry on skin samples could give informations on Ki67 and p27 kip1 expression in the skin during treatment, which is probably the reflect of 'what's going on'in the tumor.

Epidermal growth factor reception (EGFR) inhibitors have become an essential part of the standard treatment for many types of cancers such as colorectal, head and neck, lung, breast, pancreatic, sarcoma, ovarian, oesophageal and renal carcinoma.

EGFR is mainly expressed in the basal layer of the skin, where it enhances epidermal growth and wound healing and mediates an inhibition of differentiation.

However, as it is expressed in many solid tumors, its therapeutic blockade, even if beneficial for the patient, can't have no consequence on the epidermis.

The dermatologic effects of the anti-EGFR can be considered from two points of view:

I. The clinical side effects, that can be severe or even life threatening and their management – Dermatopathologic aspects will be considered.
II. The dermatologic reaction that could be considered as a simple, visual grading of the efficiency of the drug allowing discriminating potent "responders" to the other ones.

I. CLINICAL CUTANEOUS SIDE EFFECTS

In their review in 2006, Agero et al [1] have shown the pattern of adverse skin reactions to anti EGFR.

1. *Pustular eruption*: the rash resembles acne but in its pustular form, without comedones.

    It usually appears within one to three weeks after onset of treatment. This reaction is reversible. Complete resolution is usually achieved within 4 weeks of withdrawal from treatment.

    It's the most common side effect as its incidence varies from trial to trial between 60 and 80 %.

    It seems that the occurrence of the rash is more frequent with cetuximab than with gefitinib [2].

    Histology: biopsy specimens show two major patterns [2,3, 4, 5].
    -   a moderate superficial infiltrate surrounding ectatic follicular infundibula in the upper part of the follicle
    -   A superficial neutrophilic suppurative folliculitis. Special staining is usually positive for fungus or bacteria in classical acne but negative in anti-EGFR reactions.

    Immunochemistry:

    The cyclin – dependant kinase (CDK) inhibitor, p 27 Kip 1 is a negative growth regulator. It is increased in gefitinib, erlotinib and cetuximab – treated patients [6, 7, 8].

    A two fold increase of p 27 kip 1 labelling has been observed in epidermal keratinocytes in patients treated with cetuximab compared to untreated skin, especially in the basal and suprabasal kératinocytes [5].

    Ki67 expression is decreased in the epidermal basal layers, indicating a significant inhibition of cell proliferation [9, 10, 11].

    Management:
    -   topical antiseptics and antibiotics.
    -   Systemic antibiotics
    -   Topical retinoids.

2. *Abnormalities of hair growth:*

    Trichomegaly or "wavy" hair phenotype can occur during anti-EGFR treatment.

    The CDK inhibitor p 27 kip 1 appears to be involved in the differentiation of follicular epithelial cells [12].

    The down regulation of some effectors (TGF α) but synergism with others (FGF-5) results in longer hair phenotype [13].

    Management: no.

3. *Paronychia and fissuring*:

    This peculiar granuloma of the nail is not so rare as its incidence is 6 – 12 %.

    It never requires treatment withdrawal but can be very persistent.

    Management: local care.

4. *Hypersensitivity reactions:*

They have been reported with cetuximab [13, 14] EMD 72 000, [24], this gefitinib [15] and CI – 1033 [16] but not with the mAB ABX – EGF [17]. They are easy to control with anti-histamines

Management: anti-histamines.

II. ANTI-EGFR DERMATOLOGIC REACTION AS A MARKER OF ANTITUMORAL EFFICIENCY

Pharmacokinetic studies have shown that the rash parallels saturation of receptor clearance [18], which is an indirect measure of effective receptor saturation and therefore surely an indication of optimum biologic dose.

But questions remain:

Why one third of patients don't develop skin reaction, even at a very high dose?

The network of EGFR includes seven ligands and four related receptors, representing one of the most complex signalling systems in biology.

In that context, pharmacokinetic and pharmacodynamic differences can be easily imagined as well as EGFR polymorphisms among patients.

On the other hand, it has been shown that for cetuximab, ABX – EGF, erlotinib and gefinitib, rash occurs more frequently in responders [19].

Patients with at least grade 2 rash (i.e. rash with associated symptoms as pruritus or desquamation or lesions covering less than 50 % of BSA) were found to have a statistically significant improvement in tumor response [20].

Significant correlation between occurrence of rash and increased survival has also been found [14].

The situation is still more complicated than it appears at first glance e.g. as for gefinitib, the link between rash and treatment response has been shown less consistent.

On the basis of these findings, different attitudes could be proposed:

- It could be suggested that agents be used at maximal tolerated doses to maximum clinical benefit [21, 22].
- A scale of grading could be imagined concerning the clinical skin reaction as an indication of the most likely effective doses on one hand and of the maximal tolerated one on the other.
- It would make sense to relate length of exposure to likelihood of rash development : rash, as a time dependent variable and regardless of severity, has been shown to be a significant predictor of survival.
- In terms of dermatopathology, among patients having a skin reaction - suggesting that their EGFR phenotype and their EGFR pharmacokinetics and pharmacodynamics authorise to parallel their tumor and their skin – a histological scale would be needed:
  - It could consist of a quantitative measure of Ki67 expression in affected skin in comparison with unaffected one, which could provide a scale of efficiency of anti-EGFR in these patients.

– Similarly, a matched measure of expression of p 27 kip 1 in normal and affected skin could also provide information on "what's going on in the tumor".

In conclusion, if visual severity of the rash can provide very important information in terms of which doses to use, simple skin biopsies could probably provide more biological information on the efficiency of the drug.

REFERENCES

[1]   Agero A.L. et al. Dermatologic side effects associated with the epidermal growth factor receptor inhibitors. *J. Am. Acad. Dermatol.* 2006; 55 (4): 657 – 670.

[2]   Jacot W. et al. Acneiform eruption induced by epidermal growth factor receptor inhibitors in patients with solid tumors. *Br. J. Dermatol.* 2004; 151: 238 – 41.

[3]   Cohen R. et al. Safety profile of the monoclonal antibody (Mo Ab) IMC – C225, an anti-epidermal growth factor receptor (EGFR) used in the treatment of EGFR – positive tumors. *Proc. Am. Soc. Clin. Oncol.* 2000; 19: 474 a

[4]   Hidalgo M. et al. Phase I and pharmacologic study of OSI – 774, an epidermal growth factor tyrosine kinase inhibitor, in patients with advanced solid malignancies. *J. Clin. Oncol.* 2001; 19: 3267 – 79.

[5]   Busam K.J. et al. Cutaneous side-effects in cancer patients treated with anti epidermal growth factor receptor antibody C225. *Br. J. Dermatol.* 2001; 144: 1169 – 76.

[6]   Topley GI et al. P 21 (WAF 1 / lip 1) functions as a suppressor of malignant skin tumor formation and a determinant of kératinocyte stem-cell potential. *Proc. Natl. Acad. Sci USA.* 1999; 96: 9089 – 94.

[7]   Mitsui S. et al. Structure and hair follicle-specific expression of genes encoding the rat high sulphur protein B2 family. *Gene.* 1998; 208: 123 – 9.

[8]   Kijokawa H. et al. Enhanced growth of mice lacking the cyclin-dependent kinase inhibitor function of p 27 (kip 1). *Cell.* 1996; 85: 721 – 32.

[9]   Herbst RS et al. Selective oral epidermal growth factor receptor tyrosine kinase inhibitor ZD1839 is generally well tolerated and has activity in non small-cell lung cancer and other solid tumors: results of a phase I trial. *J. Clin. Oncol.* 2002; 20: 3815 – 25.

[10]   Van Hoefer U. et al. Phase I study of the humanized anti epidermal growth factor receptor monoclonal antibody EMD 72 000 in patients with advanced solid tumors that express the epidermal growth factor receptor. *J. Clin. Oncol.* 2004; 22: 175 – 84.

[11]   Albanell J. et al. Pharmacodynamic studies of the epidermal growth factor receptor inhibitor ZD1839 in skin from cancer patients: histopathologic and molecular consequences of receptor inhibition. *J. Clin. Oncol.* 2002; 20: 110 – 24.

[12]   Motzer RJ et al. Phase II trial of anti epidermal growth factor receptor antibody C225 in patients with advanced renal cell carcinoma. *Invest. New Drugs.* 2003; 21: 99 – 101.

[13]   Bence AR et al. Phase I pharmacokinetic studies evaluating single and multiple doses of oral GW572016, a dual EGFR – Erb B2 inhibitor, in healthy subjects. *Invest. New Drugs.* 2005; 23: 39 – 49.

[14]   Saltz LB et al. Phase II trial of Cetuximab in patients with refractory colorectal cancer that expresses the epidermal growth factor receptor. *J. Clin. Oncol.* 2004; 22: 1201 – 8.

[15] Ranson M et al. ZD 1839, a selective oral epidermal growth factor receptor-tyrosine kinase inhibitor, is well tolerated and active in patients with solid, malignant tumors: results of a phase I trial. *J. Clin. Oncol.* 2002; 20: 2240 – 50.

[16] Rinehart JJ et al. A phase I clinical and pharmacokinetic (PK)/food effect study on oral CI-1033, a pan-erb B tyrosine kinase inhibitor, in patients with advanced solid tumors. *Proc. Am. Soc. Clin. Oncol.* 2003; 22: 205.

[17] Rowinsky EK. Safety, pharmacokinetics and activity of ABX – EGF, a fully human anti-epidermal growth factor receptor monoclonal antibody in patients with metastatic renal cancer. *J. Clin. Oncol.* 2004; 22: 3003 – 15.

[18] Roskos L. et al. Low pharmacokinetic variability facilitates optimal dosing of ABX – EGF in cancer patients. *Proc. Am. Soc. Clin. Oncol.* 2002; 21: 1.

[19] Park J. et al. Gefitinib immunotherapy as a salvage specimen for previously treated advanced non-small lung cancer. *Clin. Cancer. Res.* 2004; 10: 4383 – 8.

[20] Vancutsem E et al. Correlation of acne rash and tumor response with Cetuximab monotherapy in patients with colorectal cancer refractory to both irinotecab and oxaliplatin. *Eur. J. Cancer. Suppl.* 2004; 2: 85.

[21] Brewer CJ et al. Phase II trial of erlotinib with temozolomide and radiation therapy in patients with newly – diagnosed glioblastoma multiforme. *J. Clin. Oncol.* 2005; 23 (suppl): 165.

[22] Mita CA et al. A pilot, pharmacokinetic and pharmacodynamic study to determine the feasibility of intra patient dose escalation to tolerate rash and the activity of maximal doses of erlotinib in previously treated patients with advanced non-small cell lung cancer. *J. Clin. Oncol.* 2005; 23: 3045.

In: Handbook of Skin Care in Cancer Patients   ISBN: 978-1-61668-419-8
Editors: Pierre Vereecken and Ahmad Awada   © 2012 Nova Science Publishers, Inc.

Chapter 9

THE COMMON AND THE UNUSUAL PRESENTATION OF SKIN METASTASES IN CANCER PATIENTS

Wolfram Fink[1] and Dirk Schadendorf[2]
[1]Hu-Brugmann, Brussels, Belgium
[2]University Hospital, Essen, Germany

ABSTRACT

Cutaneous metastases are an infrequent sign of advanced internal malignancies but may in some cases be the first opportunity to diagnose a so far unapparent cancer. Their early detection may significantly accelerate the initiation of a stage related therapy for a potentially treatable cancer. Moreover may these skin metastases serve as an easily accessible source of tumor cells in the era of adapted and specific tumor therapy. Virtually any body site can be involved, but more common sites of cutaneous metastasis are the scalp, umbilicus, chest wall, and abdominal wall. Uncommon findings are metastases to the nail bed, eye-lid, scars or benign skin lesions. The typical presentation are painless nodules, but mimicry of other cutaneous disorders has hampered diagnosis in many cases. Frequencies of cutaneous metastasis roughly correspond to the overall incidence of the various visceral malignancies, with carcinomas of the lung, breast, colon, and melanoma leading. But basically any tumor can metastasize to the skin and an exhaustive number of case reports has been published on cutaneous metastasis of rare malignancies. Even though they may occur at any time point in the course of the disease, most frequently detection of skin metastases follows the diagnosis of the primary tumor and is an ominous sign of advanced disease. Both, very early and very late metastasis to the skin has been observed, the interval between primary and metastatic diagnosis ranging from less than one week to more than twenty years. Given the therapeutic and prognostic value of an early diagnosis of cutaneous metastases, knowledge about the common and uncommon features is crucial for clinicians in charge of cancer patients.

INTRODUCTION

Cutaneous metastases not only represent a common sign of advanced internal malignancies but may in some cases be the first opportunity to diagnose a so far unapparent internal cancer [1,2]. The early detection of skin metastases may hence significantly accelerate the initiation of a stage related therapy for a potentially treatable cancer. Moreover may these skin metastases serve as an easily accessible source of tumor cells in the era of adapted and specific tumor therapy [3].

EPIDEMIOLOGY

Cutaneous metastases of internal malignancies occur infrequently, however, virtually any tumor can metastasize to the skin. For solid tumors, metastatic spread to the skin has been described with rates between 0.6% and 10% [4,5,6]. Skin metastases in leukemia and lymphoma occur with a more consistent frequency in 5 to 7% of the cases [7].

Table 1. Frequencies of cutaneous metastases by gender [1, 2b]

women		men	
breast	*69%*	*lung*	*24%*
large intestine	*9%*	*large intestine*	*19%*
malignant melanoma	*5%*	*malignant melanoma*	*13%*
ovary	*4%*	*oral squamous cell carcinoma*	*12%*
lung	4%	kidney	6%
sarcoma	2%	stomach	6%
uterine cervix	2%	esophagus	3%
pancreas	2%	sarcoma	3%
oral squamous cell carcinoma	1%	pancreas	2%
urinary bladder	1%	urinary bladder	2%
		salivary glands	2%
		breast	2%
		prostate	1%
		thyroid	1%
		liver	1%
		cutaneous squamous cell ca.	1%

Metastatic activity to the skin is not only highly tumor type specific but also gender dependent. A significant difference between the relative frequencies of cutaneous metastases in men and women can be calculated, whereas the frequencies basically correspond to those of their primary cancers. In women with skin metastases, the following distribution of the four most common primary cancers was found: breast 69%, large intestine 9%, melanoma 5%, and ovary 4% (see also table 1 and [1] and [8]). In men the four most frequent primary cancers were found as follows: lung 24%, large intestine 19%, melanoma 13%, and squamous cell carcinoma of the oral cavity 12%. The first positions in this ranking list may considerably differ in the so far published studies. This can mainly be explained by the inconsistent inclusion criteria applied in the different series published so far, as for instance the histological confirmation for skin lesions classified "metastasis" is not granted in all studies [5,6]. Moreover, the absolute and sex related frequencies of several primary cancers, such as lung cancer and melanoma, have changed considerably in the last years, and there is a need of new and histologically controlled studies to update the so far available data.

Cutaneous metastases may occur at any time point in the course of the disease, but most frequently detection of skin metastases follows the diagnosis of the primary tumor and is an ominous sign of advanced disease. Both, very early and very late metastasis to the skin has been observed.

Cutaneous metastases as the first sign of internal malignancy are termed "precocious" [1,3]. In about 21% of patients with skin metastases the primary tumor is not yet known [2]. While in men lung and kidney cancers account for the majority of precocious skin metastases, in women kidney and ovary tumors do so [2]. And due to the different absolute frequencies and incidences of these malignancies in the two genders, precocious cutaneous metastases are diagnosed about six times more often in men than in women.

Very late metastatic spread to the skin - up to 10 years after initial diagnosis of the primary cancer - has been described for breast cancers, melanomas, kidney, bladder, colon ovary and larynx [2] [Table 2].

The diagnosis of cutaneous metastatic disease is also of important prognostic value. In about 7.6% of patients skin metastases constitute the first sign of extranodal disease [5,6] and hence patient survival decreases substantially with their appearance.

Table 2. Primary tumors with typical precautious and very late presentation of cutaneous metastasis

Precautious skin metastasis	Very late skin metastasis
lung	breast
kidney	malignant melanoma
ovary	kidney
	bladder
	colon
	ovary
	larynx

ETIOLOGY OF SKIN METASTASIS

The involvement of skin in cancer disease may either be a result of the direct extension of the primary tumor or the result of a local or distant spread. For most cancerous skin lesions their type can more or less easily be defined. However, in the case of Paget's disease of breast a debate is left open on its real nature as either being a local metastasis [3] or a direct extension of its primary [5]. On the other hand, the mechanism of metastasis is undisputedly seen as a chain of multiple events, including tumor cell detachment from the primary, invasion and intravasation into a blood or lymphatic vessel, circulation, intravascular stasis, extravasation, invasion into tissue, and proliferation at the metastatic site. Moreover, different patterns of metastasis can be distinguished. One observes the distribution due to mechanical tumor stasis (leading to spread along lymphatic draining and basically in anatomic proximity), the organ or site-specific pattern, and the nonselective distribution (independent of mechanical and organ-specific factors). Further explanation for a rather unusual distribution of skin metastases may be found in models taking into account diverse physical and anatomical factors as for instance the body segmental temperature [9-12] or the role of the vertebral venous system [13-15]. The latter refers to a system of valveless veins including the epidural veins, perivertebral veins, and veins of the head and neck. This system parallels and bypasses the portal venous system, the pulmonary system, and the caval system, still keeping interconnections with them. Circulation in the vertebral venous system occurs under low pressure and may explain for example the possibility of metastasis from genitourinary tract malignancies to the head.

CLINICAL FEATURES

The Common Presentation

Many clinical appearances of cutaneous metastases have been reported so far, however, common features and localizations may be distinguished from rather unusual presentations.

For any suddenly appearing firm and non-tender nodule skin metastasis should be in the panel of differential diagnoses and a biopsy should be considered. Skin metastases usually present as aggregates of nodular lesions [5], but solitary lesions are also frequent [3]. They may appear as dermal papules or subcutaneous nodules, they may form inflammatory patches or fixed indurated lesions and they may ulcerate or form bullae [5]. The skin at the site of metastases may look inflammatory (carcinoma erysipeloides) [fig. 1], become sclerotic or be bound down (carcinoma en cuirasse). An irritated umbilical skin may be the presenting sign of skin metastasis to this site known as the Sister Mary Joseph nodule [16]. Cutaneous metastases to the scalp can cause alopecia (alopecia neoplastica) [fig. 2] and in some cases an atypical presentation of "scalp alopecia due to a clinically unapparent or minimally apparent neoplasm" (SACUMAN) [17].

Terminology of skin metastasis is very descriptive and historically linked to the observations made in breast cancer, this being a very common malignancy with a high incidence of cutaneous spread [3].

The sclerotic aspect of some type of metastatic breast cancer reminded Velpeau in 1838 of the metal breastplate of a cuirassier and he named it "cancer en cuirasse". The term "Paget's disease" honors its observer who in 1874 described a "long-persistent eczema" starting on the nipple and areola which is associated with an underlying cancer.

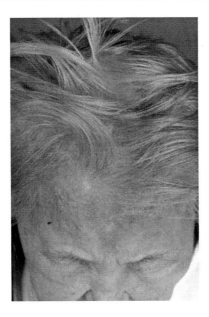

Figure 1. Carcinoma erysipeloides.

"Carcinoma erysipelatodes" was first described by Hutchinson in 1893 as "cancer erythema" or "erythema-scirrhus of the skin in association with cancer of the breast". In the same year two subtypes of the "erythema-scirrhus" the "lenticular" and the "tuberose" where described by Crocker. The "carcinoma lenticulare" corresponds to cutaneous nodules whereas "carcinoma tuberose" signifies subcutaneous nodules. In 1933 the term "carcinoma telangiectaticum" was introduced by Parkes Weber to describe a form of breast cancer showing pin-point telangiectases and dilated capillaries. Metastatic tumor nodules of the umbilicus are nowadays referred to as "Sister Mary Joseph's nodules". This term was introduced by Baily to honor Sister Mary Joseph, an assistant to Dr W.J. Mayo during the early 1900s in the Mayo Clinic, who first noted the umbilical nodules in patients with abdominal cancer [18].

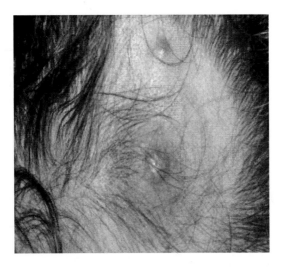

Figure 2. Alopecia neoplastica.

The particular features of cutaneous metastases from the most common primary cancers are presented in the following.

Common Sources of Cutaneous Metastases

Breast Cancer

Breast carcinoma accounts for the majority of cutaneous metastases in women (69%) and for about half of the total in both sexes. Metastases occur locally in 86%, distally in 14% and rarely as miliary disease [19]. Most common site for distant metastasis is the scalp.

Eight distinct clinical types of cutaneous involvement have been described in breast carcinoma, even though they are not limited to breast cancer but also seen in other malignancies [3].

1) The *inflammatory metastatic carcinoma* appears as erysipelas-like patches or plaques without clinical signs of acute inflammation, usually affecting the breast and adjacent skin. Capillary congestion caused by deposition of malignant cells between lymphatics and not acute inflammatory infiltrate is the basis of the inflammatory aspect of these lesions. Rarely other sites, such as the forearm only, may be involved [20]. Other malignancies sharing a similar appearance of metastatic lesions are carcinoma of the pancreas, parotid, tonsils, colon, stomach, rectum, melanoma, pelvic organs, ovary, uterus, prostate, and lung (fig. 1).

2) *Telagiectatic metastatic carcinoma* can clinically resemble the inflammatory type but more often appears as violaceous papulovesicles close to the aspect of lymphangioma circumscriptum. In some cases the aspect is pruritic and very rarely it may mimic cutaneous vasculitis. Histology is also similar to the inflammatory type but more dilated vessels and aggregates of erythrocytes and tumor cells are seen.

3) *En cuirasse metastatic carcinoma* clinically presents as a sclerodermatous and morphea-like induration of the skin. Usually lesions appear first as scattered, firm lenticular papulonodules on an erythematous or bluish cutaneous surface, later they form a confluent sclerodermoid plaque. Histology shows a highly fibrotic stroma with only few remaining tumor cells. Other malignancies with similar metastatic lesion are cancers of the lung, gastrointestinal tract, kidney and others.

4) *Nodular metastatic carcinoma* usually presents as aggregates of tender papulonodules or nodules, but sometimes only solitary lesions are found. Ulceration and bullae are possible and sometimes intense pigmentation may suggest the presence of melanoma or other pigmented tumors.

5) *Alopecia neoplastica* most probably appears through hematogenous metastasis mimicking alopecia areata by its circular areas of painless and nonpruritic alopecia. The skin of these plaques shows a red-pink and smooth surface [2] and sometimes clinical appearance is closely resembling the image of lupus erythematosus, lichen planopilaris, pseudopelade, or morpheaform basal cell carcinoma. Alopecia neoplastica can be the presenting sign of metastatic breast cancer, thus, breast examination and skin biopsies from the alopecic lesion should be considered [3].

6) *Paget's disease of the breast* presents as an erythematous patch or plaque with sharp borders and scaling in the area of the nipple or the areola and is almost always

associated with an underlying breast cancer. It may also occur in men and appear on basis of an ectopic breast tissue or a supernumerary nipple. Prognosis of the disease is dependent on the presence or absence of a palpable tumor and a concomittand adenopathy. It may occur together with other types of cutaneous breast metastases and remains associated to underlying breast cancer, even if it clinically "healed" [21].

7) *Breast carcinoma of the inframammary crease* appears as an exophytic cutaneous nodule and may due to its aspect be mistaken as a primary cutaneous basal or squamous cell carcinoma [22]. More frequently seen in women with pendulous breasts it may be confounded with intertriginous dermatitis.

8) *Histioid metastastic breast carcinoma of the eyelid* has been described in a few patients [23] and appears as painless nodules, diffuse eyelid swelling, or ulcerative lesions of both upper and lower eyelids. Solitary nodules are often mistaken clinically for chalazia.

Extramammary Paget's Disease

Morphology and histology being similar to Paget's disease of the breast, the predilection sites of these lesions are the axilla, the external ear canal, the eyelids, or the anogenital region, then easily mistaken as an intertriginous dermatitis [fig. 3]. Three types of extramammary Paget's disease are known: the *first type* unassociated with an underlying cancer, the *second* in association with an underlying apocrine or ecrine gland carcinoma, and the *third type* associated with another malignancy, usually cancers of the gastrointestinal of genitourinary tract. In some cases more than one site of predilection may be involved.

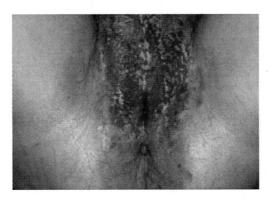

Figure 3. Extramammary Paget's disease.

Lung Cancer

In men a primary in the lung is the most common source of cutaneous metastases (24%). Predilection sites for metastasis are the chest wall and the posterior abdomen, but they can appear on any part of the skin. Small cell carcinoma of the lung was observed to characteristically spread to the skin of the back [5]. The general appearance of cutaneous metastases is a localized cluster of nodules. Their aspect has also been described as more vascular, zosteriform or as carcinoma erysipelatodes. Rarely, they appear at the site of thoracostomy, in a needle aspiration tract, or at the site of a burn scar [24,25].

Carcinoma of the Large Intestines

In both women and men, rectum and colon carcinoma are the second most common primaries of metastasis to the skin, the majority of cutaneous metastasis originating from the rectum [3]. Most common is the involvement of the abdominal wall with tendency to scars [1] and the inguinal and perineal region. Distant skin metastases have also been described on scalp and face [26-29]. Metastases may appear clinically as inflammatory carcinoma in the groins, in the supraclavicular area, on the neck, or on the face. Forms of grouped vascular nodules in the inguinal folds and on the scrotum [29] as well as sessile or pedunculated nodules on the buttocks have been described [30]. Hidradenitis suppurativa may be the misleading diagnosis when nodular and inflamed metastases appear in the perianal region [6].

Melanoma

Melanoma is the third most common source of skin metastases in women and men [1,8]. Both, cutaneous and extracutaneous melanomas metastasize to the skin [1,6,8] where they usually appear as multiple and disseminated strongly pigmented but sometimes also amelanotic nodules with no particular predilection site (fig. 4). Sometimes one or two of these nodules may become particularly large [3]. When the first cutaneous metastases are detected, usually also visceral metastases are present, this being an ominous sign of advanced stage of disease [31]. Melanoma is one of the most common malignancies associated with metastatic disease to the mucosal surfaces of the gastrointestinal tract and even though rare, metastases to the upper aerodigestive tract are reported [32, 33]. Thus, regular inspection of the visible oral mucosa should be included in the follow up of these patients (fig. 5).

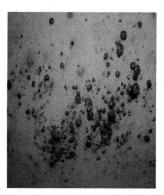

Figure 4. Melanoma metastases.

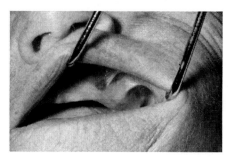

Figure 5. Mucosal metastasis.

Squamous Cell Carcinomas of the Oral Cavity

Squamous cell carcinomas of the oral cavity are the fourth most common source of skin metastases in men (12%) but only a rare one in women (1%) [8]. Cutaneous metastases usually appear in sun-damaged skin of the head and neck and may sometimes be indistinguishable, clinically and histologically, from primary cutaneous squamous cell carcinomas [8]. Usually a primary tumor has already been diagnosed when the first metastases appear.

Ovarian Tumors

Gynecological malignancies only rarely metastasize to the skin, *carcinoma of the ovary* being the most common with 3.5% of the patients developing cutaneous metastases [34]. But they are the fourth most common source of cutaneous metastases in women. Skin metastases are frequently found to be the presenting sign of the disease [3]. Predilection sites are the abdominal skin, particularly the umbilicus [6,12, 34], the trunk and the back. They also tend to occur on scars and on sites of paracentesis [34]. Particular clinical forms such as herpetiform lesions [36], inflammatory and erysipelas-like metastases [37] or lymphatic carcinomatosis resembling scleroderma have been described [38].

Carcinoma of the Uterine Cervix

Carcinoma of the uterine cervix only accounts for about 2% of skin metastases in women [8, 39]. Cutaneous metastases appear as plaques, nodules, carcinoma telangiectaticum or as inflammatory patches and plaques. Most commonly metastases are found on the abdominal skin, the vulva, the anterior chest wall, the lower extremities, and the scalp [34, 40, 41].

Endometrial Cancer

Contrary to endometriosis, a benign form of metastasizing ovarian disease where nodules are frequently found in the umbilicus and in surgical scars, cutaneous metastases of the malignant endometrial cancer are rare [8]. They can appear as multiple or solitary subcutaneous nodules on the scalp, the trunk, and the legs, rarely in abdominal surgical scars.

Renal Cell Carcinomas

Showing a tendency to either precocious or very late cutaneous metastases, renal cell carcinomas are a common source of surprise [1, 2]. They represent the fourth most common source for skin metastases [8]. Cutaneous metastases clinically appear as solitary or widespread nodules in blue, violaceus or flesh color, sometimes showing a strong vascularity. Rarely they may present as a cutaneous horn [42, 43]. Predilection sites are the head and the neck where tumor cells seem to spread easily via the vertebral venous system [44]. Trunk and extremities may also be sites of cutaneous metastases.

Gastric Adenocarcinoma

Cutaneous metastases from gastric adenocarcinoma account for about 6% of skin metastases in men [8]. They show a large variety of clinical presentations, from nonspecific nodules to zosteriform or erysipelas-like lesions, sometimes forming scarring alopecia. They may mimic epidermoid kysts, condyloma acuminatum, or benign soft tissue tumors. Appearance at the site of a congenital melanocytic nevus [45, 46] or at the site of a percutaneous endoscopic gastrostomy has been described [47]. Sites of predilection are the head, eyebrow, neck, axilla, chest, finger and umbilicus [8, 48-50].

Lymphomas and Leukemias

Cutaneous metastases in patients with leukemia and lymphoma have been reported in 5-7% of the cases and are more common than skin metastases in melanoma patients [4,7]. Distinction between primary and metastatic lymphoma of the skin may be difficult but is of high importance, particularly when the question comes to whether it is a primary or secondary cutaneous CD30+ large cell lymphoma or a non-Hodgkin's B-cell lymphoma.

Clinically, skin metastases in both, *Hodgkin's and non –Hodgkin's lymphomas* present either as erythematous or violaceous plaques or nodules of variable size. They have a firm consistency, may sometimes form large plaques termed "lymphoma en cuirasse" [51], and can - when of bigger size - ulcerate and form deep lesions. Forms resembling erythema nodosum have been reported [52] as well as cutaneous infiltrations from underlying involved lymph nodes or via retrograde spreading from affected lymph nodes [53].

Cutaneous infiltrates from *leukemia* show a variety of lesions such as macules, papules, nodules, plaques, ecchymoses, palpable purpura or ulcerations [54]. In several subtypes of leukemia very specific infiltrates are found:

In *congenital leukemia* children may present as "blueberry muffin babies", a term also used in congenital neuroblastoma [55, 56]. The aspect of disseminated blue, red, or violaceous and firm nodules explains this term. These infiltrates are usually preceding other manifestations of the leukemia by several months.

Only *chronic lymphocytic leukemia* has so far presented with erythrodermic and bullous lesions [54].

Granulocytic leukemia has a predilection to the trunk with multiple large cutaneous tumors [57, 58].

Acute myelocytic leukemia may develop cutaneous lesions called "myeloblatomas" or "granulocytic sarcomas" which change their color into green when myeloperoxidase levels in leukemia cells rise. They are then termed "chloromas" [54].

Myelomonocytic leukemia may present with pernio-like plaques on the extremities of fingers and nose [59].

Monocytic leukemia shows typical involvement of skin and mucous tissues with violacious papules or nodules (fig. 6) that may ulcerate or form bullae and with gingival infiltrations [54, 60, 61].

In *adult T-cell leukemia* skin metastases appear in up to 75% of the patients, independent of the subtype. The large variety of lesions comprises maculopapules, plaques and large and ulcerative tumors.

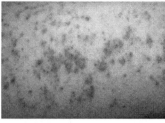

Figure 6. Skin involvement of leukemia.

Neuroblastoma

Congenital neuroblastoma is the most common cancer found at birth and cutaneous metastasis occurs in 32% of the cases [56]. The typical clinical appearance of skin metastases as widespread firm but nontender subcutaneous nodules of bluish or violaceous color has given rise to the term "blueberry muffin baby". A typical blanching for up to 1 hour is observed, when the lesions are stroke, this phenomenon being explained by catecholamine release from the tumor cells causing vasoconstriction.

Predilection Sites

Although metastatic spread may involve any site of the skin, a predilection for certain body regions can be observed among the different tumor types [3, 6, 62] [fig. 7].

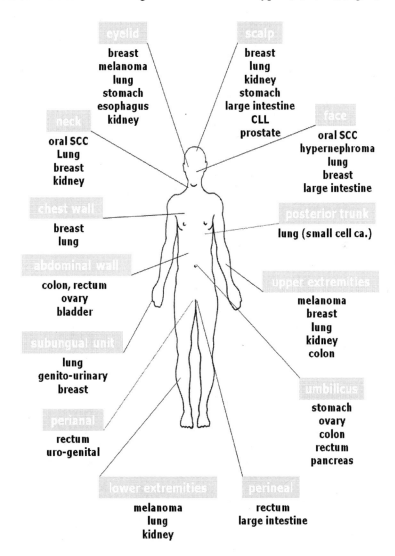

Figure 7. Predilection sites of skin metastases.

Knowledge of predilection sites can particularly be helpful in clinical practice, when skin metastases are the presenting sign of systemic disease and when histology of a first biopsy remains inconclusive due to a lack of differentiation and the loss of characteristic immunohisto-chemical staining frequently observed among skin metastases of adenocarcinomas [1].

In about 75% of male patients with cutaneous metastases sites of metastasis are limited to the head, neck, anterior chest, and abdomen, altogether accounting for only 25% of the body surface [62]. In about 75% of female patients with cutaneous metastases the lesions are limited to the anterior chest and abdomen, accounting for even less than 20% of the skin surface [62].

Metastases to the facial skin most often come from squamous cell carcinomas of the oral cavity, hypernephromas, lung cancer, and breast cancer [3]. Cutaneous metastases to the neck most often are direct extensions from cervical lymph nodes invaded by lung cancer, breast cancer, or squamous cell carcinoma of the oral cavity. Rarer sites of cutaneous metastases are the upper and lower extremities, melanoma, breast, lung, kidney, and colon cancer being the primaries reported for the upper extremities and melanoma, lung, and kidney for the lower extremities [62].

The scalp and the umbilicus are the most common sites for metastases and deserve a more detailed description.

Scalp Metastases

The scalp is the predilection site for metastases from a variety of primary tumors. In women breast cancer is most frequently reported as the source, whereas in men lung cancer and kidney cancer account for the majority of scalp metastases [62]. Other malignancies also diagnosed with scalp metastases are large intestinal cancers, gastric cancer, renal cell carcinoma, prostate cancer, and leukaemia [3, 19]. Cutaneous metastases to the scalp appear as nodules and plaques and may be the primary cause of alopecia (alopecia neoplastica) [2, 63, 64]. Sometimes the infiltration of metastatic cells is not florid but nevertheless destroys the hair follicles. The alopecia is then termed SACUMAN ("scalp alopecia due to a clinically unapparent or minimally apparent neoplasm") [17]. In one case of metastatic breast cancer scalp erythema without alopecia was observed [65].

Umbilical Metastases or the "Sister Mary Joseph's Nodule"

Umbilical metastases account for about 10% of all metastases to the abdominal wall [48]. The majority of the Sister Mary Joseph's nodules are adenocarcinomas originating from intra-abdominal organs [48-50]. The most common primaries are carcinomas of the stomach, ovary, colon, rectum and pancreas. Rarer and unusual primaries for Sister Mary Joseph's nodules are renal cell carcinomas [66] and prostate carcinoma [67]. Clinically, umbilical metastases appear as firm and indurated plaques or nodules, accompanied by visible vascularisation. In some cases discharges from fissures or ulcerations may be seen. Usually umbilical metastases appear in the late stage of systemic malignancy , but in some case studies [48] they are the presenting lesion of internal malignancy in more than 40% of the patients. Most patients die within months after the appearance of umbilical metastases due to extensive metastasis [66-68]. This rapid tumor cell spread is seen in the context of a hematogenous spread and a direct extension, favored by the potential anatomical connections between the umbilicus and the portal system, the lateral thoracic and internal mammary veins which might serve as routes for a rapid tumor cells dissemination.

THE UNUSUAL PRESENTATION

An unusual presentation of skin metastases may be a matter of surprise and of a delayed diagnosis. Primary tumors which frequently metastasize to the skin may show skin involvement of untypical morphology and in unusual location. And one may come across neoplastic skin lesions which in histopathological examination turn out to be metastases of primary cancers rarely metastasizing to the skin.

Rare Sources of Cutaneous Metastases

Esophageal Cancer
Cutaneous metastases from esophageal cancer are rather rare (3% of skin metastases in men) [8]. Independent of the different histological types, adenocarcinoma, squamous cell carcinoma, mucoepidermoid carcinoma, or small-cell carcinoma, clinical appearance of skin metastases is quite uniform as single or multiple cutaneous nodules [39].

Sarcomas
Literally all sarcoma types, leiomyosarcoma, rhabdomyosarcoma, fibrosarcoma, malignant fibrous histiocytoma, chondrosarcoma, Ewing's sarcoma, osteogenic sarcoma and undifferentiated sarcomas may metastasize to the skin, but they are a rare source of cutaneous metastases in women and men (2-3%) [8]. They have shown generalized cutaneous metastasis as well as localized lesions including the scalp.

Pancreatic Cancer
Skin metastases from pancreatic cancer are rare and represent only 2% of all cutaneous metastases in men and women [8]. Metastases from gastrin-producing cells are exceptional, non-islet-cell adenocarcinomas account for the majority of cutaneous metastases, which are mainly located in the umbilicus [8, 47, 69, 70].

Cancers of the Urinary Tract
Cutaneous metastases from *bladder cancer* account for only 1-2% of skin metastases in women and men respectively [8]. Other primaries in the urinary tract as sources for cutaneous metastases are transitional cell carcinomas of the *renal pelvis* and *urethra* [71]. General clinical presentation are intradermal nodules with predilection to the umbilicus and inguinal folds [39]. Rare presentations such as zosteriform skin lesions [72] or papilomatous lesions [73] in the urethra have been described.

Cancers of the Salivary Glands
Only 2% of cutaneous metastases in men and 1% in women originate from cancers of salivary glands [8]. Metastases have been observed on the scalp, the face, or on the eyelid and

different aspects, such as nodules, inflammatory plaques or even kerion have been reported [74, 75].

Prostate Cancer

Only 1% of cutaneous metastases in men are due to prostate cancer [8]. They may appear as red or violaceous nodules, mimic pyoderma, show zosteriform lesions, and when they appear on the scalp, they may be mistaken as pilar kysts [76-79]. Typically, metastases are found in the inguinal area, on the penis, on the lower abdominal skin, or on the thighs.

Thyroid Cancers

Independent of their histological origin, medullary, follicular, and papillary thyroid carcinoma are all reported to metastasize to the skin, but to an altogether low frequency of only 1% of all cutaneous metastases in men [8]. Cutaneous metastases present as nodules, mainly on the abdomen but they have also been reported on the face and on the scalp.

Liver Cancers

Hepatocellular carcinoma (HCC) as the most common primitive malignant liver tumor only rarely metastasizes to the skin (1% of skin metastases in men) [8]. The most common locations of skin metastases are the face and the scalp. They appear there as unique or multiple, reddish and firm, painless nodules of 1-5 cm in diameter [80]. Usually, ulceration is not observed but sometimes they may appear as necrotic and purulent lesions [81] or, on the other hand, they may have a hemangiomatous morphology [82] that can easily lead to profuse bleeding when incised or injured surgically. The presence of cutaneous metastases from HCC as the first sign of onset is very unusual [80] as is the location on the eyelid, reported in combination in one patient [83].

Cutaneous Squamous Cell Carcinoma

Skin metastases from cutaneous squamous cell carcinoma are rare (1% of skin metastases in men) [8] and it may even histologically be difficult to distinguish between metastasis and primary cutaneous tumor [84]. Primary tumors in high risk locations, such as mucocutaneous surfaces (penis and vulva) and osteomyelitic scars display cutaneous metastases more frequently [3].

Cancers of the upper Respiratory Tract

Nasopharyngeal, laryngeal, and tracheal cancers and their cutaneous metastases are mainly squamous cell carcinomas. Among skin metastases from laryngeal primaries also adenocarcinomas and carcinoid tumors are described [85]. Clinically, cutaneous metastases appear as solitary or multiple nodules with variable localizations, such as trunk, scalp, face, and extremities. Nasopharyngeal cancer has repeatedly been reported to metastasize to the penis [86].

Other Tumors

In some studies of cutaneous metastatic disease, metastases of unkown primaries, the so called "cancer of unknown primary" (CUP) rank in fourth position among the most frequent skin metastases [5].

The complete number of tumors having been reported with cutaneous metastasis is exhaustive, therefore only a few more examples will be mentioned here. Among the rare carinoid tumors, which appear in various organs and anatomic localizations, cutaneous metastases from tumors in the bronchi are reported as the most frequent ones [3]. Other tumors are neuroendocrine tumors from different sites, adenocarcinomas of the gall bladder, the fallopian tube, and the vulva, pheochromocytomas, teratocarcinomas, testicular or placental choriocarcinomas, testicular seminomas and Leydig cell tumors, adrenal cortical adenocarcinomas, malignant ameloblastomas, atrial myxomas, chordomas, thymomas, brain tumors, and not to forget cutaneous appendageal tumors.

Uncommon Clinical Presentation of Cutaneous Metastases

For many types of cancer mimicry of other cutaneous disorders has been reported when they metastasize to the skin (sebaceous or pilar cysts, pyogenic granuloma, herpes zoster, Kaposi's sarcoma, alopecia areata, lymphangioma, morphea, kerion, keratoacanthoma, hidradenitis suppurativa, and many others) [table 3]. Therefore, cutaneous metastasis should always be included in the differential diagnosis of such cutaneous lesions.

Table 3. Cutaneous metastases simulating other cutaneous disorders

Primary skin disorder	Primary malignancy
"Blueberry muffin baby" (viral)	Neuroblastoma, congenital leukemia
Multiple cylindromas	Prostate
Sebaceous or pilar cysts	Prostate, rarely colon or breast
Pyogenic granuloma	Renal cell
Kaposi's sarcoma	Renal, cervix
Alopecia areata	Breast
Lymphangiomas	Breast, rarely lung, cervix, ovary
Morphea	Breast, rarely stomach,lung, mixed tumor,lacrimal gland
Erysipelas	Breast (inflammatory type), rarely others
Primary skin cancer, inflammatory fold	Breast
Chancre	Lymphoma, nasopharyngeal transitional cell
Gumma	Lymphoma
Kerion	Salivary gland adenocarcinoma
Primary skin tumors of head and neck	Paranasal sinus tumors
Keratoacanthoma	Breast cancer
Hidradenitis suppurativa	Rectal adenocarcinoma

From Schwartz RA. Cutaneous metastatic disease. *J Am Acad Dermatol.* 1995.

Uncommon Sites of Metastasis to the Skin

Metastasis to the Subungual Unit

Metastases under the nail bed are infrequent events but when they occurred they were the first sign of a previously unsuspected primary malignancy in nearly half of the patients [87]. Common primary tumors have their origin in the lung (41%), genitourinary system (17%, of which kidney 11%), and breast (9%). Metastatic subungual tumors predominantly involve the digits of the upper extremities, less often only the great toe is involved or a symmetrical distribution is detected. The metastases have a variable clinical appearance, but the most common morphologies are an erythematous enlargement of the distal digit or a red to violaceous nodule with distortion of the nail plate, the soft tissue or both. They are usually painful and initially mistaken as infections. Patients with subungual metastases have a poor prognosis with usually only a few months survival after diagnosis.

Metastasis to the Eyelid

Metastases to the eyelids are rare events, accounting for less than 1% of malignant eyelid lesions [88]. They have been reported as the presenting sign of internal malignancy in up to 27% of the cases. The most common primary is breast cancer with up to 50% of all eyelid metastases, making metastasis to the eyelid 3 times more frequent in women than in men. Other primary cancers are melanoma, lung, stomach, esophagus, kidney, thyroid, parotid, trachea, colon, and hepatocellular carcinoma, most of them being single case reports [88, 89]. Metastases from breast cancer commonly present as painless indurations, metastases from lung cancers as solitary nodular lesions. Other clinical presentations reported are diffuse eyelid swelling or ulcerative lesions of both upper and lower eyelids. Due to the misleading localization these metastases are often mistaken clinically for chalazia.

Predilection to Scars

Most commonly seen are the local metastases in or close to a scar after surgical cure of the primary, the so called "iatrogenic metastases". They usually appear during the first year after surgery [2]. Apart from this mechanically driven spread of tumor cells there is the observation of metastasis to unrelated surgical or traumatic scars. Such unexpected metastasis of a mostly so far undiagnosed neoplasm to scar sites is reported for breast cancer, ovarian cancer, colorectal cancer, liver cancer, oral or laryngeal cancers, renal and endometrial cancers [2, 34, 90-93]. These lesions are regularly misdiagnosed as hypertrophic scars, foreign body reactions, granulomas, neuromas, calcifications, or squamous cell carcinomas. Therefore, new nodules in old or new scars should undergo histopathological examination.

Metastasis to Preexisting Skin Lesions

Metastasis to an unrelated and preexisting skin lesion has also been reported. Cutaneous metastases to the site of melanocytic nevi have been observed with gastric carcinoma [94] and breast adenocarcinoma [95]. In another case "occult cutaneous metastasis" from a previously diagnosed breast cancer was the accidental second diagnosis in the excision biopsy of a basal cell carcinoma [96]. This latter case may serve as double example, firstly for a clinically unapparent cutaneous metastasis, and secondly for the appearance of very late skin metastases, more than 14 years after diagnosis of the breast cancer.

REFERENCES

[1]   Weedon D. In: *Skin pathology*, 2nd ed. Edinburgh: *Churchill Livingstone* 2002; p. 1046-52.

[2]   Brownstein MH, Helwig EB. Spread of tumors to the skin. *Arch Dermatol.* 1973;107:80-6.

[3]   Schwartz RA. Cutaneous metastatic disease. *J Am Acad Dermatol.* 1995 Aug;33(2 Pt 1):161-82.

[4]   Spencer PS Helm TN. Skin metastases in cancer patients. *Cutis* 1987;119-21.

[5]   Lookingbill DP, Spangler N, Helm KF. Cutaneous metastases in patients with metastatic carcinoma: a retrospective study of 4020 patients. *J Am Acad Dermatol* 1993;29:228-36.

[6]   Lookingbill D, Spangler N, SextonFM. Skin involvement as the presenting sign of internal carcinoma. A retrospective study of 7316 cancer patients.*J Am Acad Dermatol* 1990;22:19-26.

[7]   Ricevuti G, Mazzone A, Rossini S et al. Skin involvement in hemopathies: specific cutaneous manifestations of acute nonlymphoid leukaemias and non-Hodgkin lymphomas. *Dermatologica* 1985;17:250-4.

[8]   Brownstein MH, Helwig EB. Metastatic tumors of skin. *Cancer* 1972;29:1298-307.

[9]   Schürich O. Über Hautmetastase im Bestrahlungsfeld bei Pyloruscarcinom. *Z f Krebsforschung* 1934;41:47-50.

[10]   Schmidt A. Herpetische Eruptionen als Vorstadium eines Hautcarcinoms neben Herpes zoster. *Arch f Dermat u Syph* (Wien) 1904;19:321-8.

[11]   Fay T, Henry GC. Correlation of body segmental temperature and its relation to the location of carcinomatous metastasis: clinical observations and response to methods of refrigeration. *Surg Gynecol Obstet* 1938;66:512-24.

[12]   Pack GT, Booher RJ. Localization of metastatic cancer by trauma. *N Y State J Med* 1949;49:1839-41.

[13]   Batson OV. The role of the vertebral veins in metastatic processes. *Ann Intern Med* 1942;16:38-45.

[14]   Hussey HH. Skin metastasis from malignant neoplasms [Letter]. *Arch Dermatol* 1982;118:289.

[15]   Schwartz RA, Fleishman JS. Reply to Hussey [Letter]. *Arch Dermatol* 1982;118:289-90.

[16]   Powell FC, Cooper AJ, Massa MC, et al. Sister Mary Joseph's nodule: a clinical and histologic study. *J Am Dermatol* 1984.10:610-5.

[17]   Scheinfeld N. Review of Scalp Alopecia due to a clinically unapparent or minimally apparent neoplasm (SACUMAN). *Acta Derm Venereol* 2006;86:387-92.

[18]   Bailey H. Demonstration of physical signs in clinical surgery. Baltimore: Williams & Wilkins, 1960;356.

[19]   Schwartz RA. Histopathological aspects of cutaneous metastatic disease. *J Am Acad Dermatol* 1995;3:649-57.

[20]   Tschen EH, Apisamthanarax P. Inflammatory metastatic carcinoma of the breast. *Arch Dermatol* 1981;117:117:120-1.

[21] Masters RK, Robertson JFR, Blamey RW. Healed Paget's disease of the nipple [Letter]. *Lancet* 1993;341:253.

[22] Watson JR, Watson CG. Carcinoma of the mammary crease: a neglected clinical entitiy. *JAMA* 1969;209:1718-9.

[23] Hood CI, Front RL, Zimmerman LE. Metastatic mammary carcinoma in the eyelid with histiocytoid appearance. *Cancer* 1973;31:793-800.

[24] HazelriggDE, Rudolph AH. Inflammatory metastatic carcinoma: carcinoma erysipelatoides. *Arch Dermatol* 1977;113:69-70.

[25] Balakrishnan C, Noorily MJ, Prasad JK, et al. Metastatic adenocarcinoma in a recent burn scar. *Burns* 1994;20:371-2.

[26] Nishitani K, Nishitani H, Shimoda Y. Cutaneous invasion of mucinous andenocarcinoma of the appendix. *J Dermatol* 1987;14:167-9.

[27] Gmitter TL, Dhawan SS, Philips MG, et al. Cutaneous metastases of colonic adenocarcinoma. *Cutis* 1990;46:66-8.

[28] Lee M, Duke EE, Munoz J, et al. Colorectal cancer presenting with a cutaneous metastatic lesion on the scalp. *Cutis* 1995;55:37-8.

[29] Nazzari G, Drago F, Malatto M, et al. Epidermoid anal canal carcinoma metastatic to the sin: a clinical mimic of prostate adenocarcinoma metastases. *J Dermatol Surg Oncol* 1994;20:765-6.

[30] Wiener K. Skin manifestations of internal disordes (dermadromes). St Louis: CV Mosby, 1947:810-5.

[31] Patel JK, Didolkar MS, Pickren JW, et al. Metastatic pattern of malignant melanoma: a study of 216 autopsy cases. *Am J Surg* 1978;135:807-10.

[32] Henderson LT, Robbins KT, Weitzner S: Upper aerodigestive tract metastases in disseminated malignant melanoma. *Arch Otolaryngol Head Neck Surg* 1986;112:659-663.

[33] Fink W, Zimpfer A, Ugurel S. Mucosal metastases in malignant melanoma. *Onkologie* 2003;26:249-251.

[34] Dauplat J, Hacker NF, Nieberg RK, et al. Distant metastases in epithelial ovarian carcinoma. *Cancer* 1987;60:1561-6.

[35] Cormio G, Capotorto M, Di Vango G, et al. Skin metastases in ovarian carcinoma: a report of nine cases and review of the literature. *Gynec Oncol* 2003;90:682-5.

[36] Eckman I, Brodkin RH, Rickert RR. Cutaneous metastases from carcinoma of the ovary. *Cutis* 1994;54:348-50.

[37] Lever LR, Holt PJA. Carcinoma erysipeloides. *Br J Dermatol* 1991;124:279-82.

[38] Diel IJ, Kühn W, Kaufmann M, et al. Lymphangiosis carcinomatosa der Haut beim Ovarialkarzinom unter dem klinischen Bild einer Sklerodermie. *Geburtshilfe Frauenheilkd* 1991;51:572-3.

[39] Brady LW, O'Neill EA, Farber SH. Unusual sites of metastases. *Semin Oncol* 1977;4:59-64.

[40] Imachi M, Tsukamoto N, Kinoshita S, et al. Skin metastasis from carcinoma of the uterine cervix. *Gynecol Oncol* 1993;48:349-54.

[41] Hayes AG, Berry AD III. Cutaneous metastasis from squamous cell carcinoma of the cervix. *J Am Acad Dermatol* 1992;26:846-50.

[42] Peterson JL, McMarlin SL. Metastatic renal-cell carcinoma presenting as a cutaneous horn. *J Dermatol Surg Oncol* 1983;9:815-8.

[43] Cuckow P, Doyle D. Renal cell carcinoma presenting in the skin. *J R Soc Med* 1991;84:497-8.

[44] Lumpkin III LR, Tschen JA. Renal cell carcinoma metastatic to the skin. *Cutis* 1984;34:143-4.

[45] Hartschuh W, Bersch A. Hautmetastasen eines Magenkarzinoms unter dem Bild eines benignen mesenchymalen Tumors. *Hautarzt* 1981;32:476-8.

[46] Betke M, Süss R, Hohenleutner U, et al. Gastric carcinoma metastatic to the site of a congenital melanocytic nevus. *J Am Acad Dermatol* 1993;28:866-9.

[47] Schiano TD, Pfister D, Harrison L, et al. Neoplastic seeding as complication of percutaneous endscopic gastrostomy. *Am J Gastroenterol* 1994;89:131-3.

[48] Steck WD, Helwig EB. Tumors of the umbilicus. *Cancer* 1965; 18:907.

[49] Barrow MV. Metastatic tumors of the umbilicus. *J Chronic Dis* 1966; 19: 1113.

[50] Powell FC, Cooper AJ, Massa MC, Goellner JR, Su WPD. Sister Mary Joseph's nodule: a clinical and histological study. *J Am Acad Dermatol* 1984; 10:610.

[51] Park KD, Kim YK, Chun SI. Lymphoma en cuirasse. *J Am Acad Dermatol* 1995;32:519-20.

[52] Matsuoka LY. Neoplastic erythema nodosum. *J Am Acad Dermatol* 1995;32:316-63.

[53] Benninghoff DL, Medina A, Alexander LL, et al. The mode of spread of Hodgkin's disease to the skin. *Cancer* 1970;26:1135-40.

[54] Su WPD, Buechner SA, Li C-Y. Clinicopathologic correlations in leukemia cutis. *J Am Acad Dermatol* 1984;11:121-8.

[55] Resnik KS, Brod BB. Leukemia cutis in congenital leukaemia: analysis and review of the world literature with report of an additional case. *Ach Dermatol* 1993;129:1301-6.

[56] de la Luz Orozco-Covarrubias M, Tamayo-Sanchez L, Duran McKinster C et al. Malignant cutaneous tumors in children. *J Am Acad Dermatol* 1994 ;30 :243-9.

[57] Long JC, Mihm MC. Multiple granulocytic tumors of the skin: report of six cases of myelogenous leukaemia with initial manifestations in the skin. *Cancer* 1977;39:2004-16.

[58] Ritter JH, Goldstein NS, Argenyi Z, et al. Granulocytic sarcoma: an immunohistologic comparison with peripheral T-cell lymphoma in paraffin sections. *J Cutan Pathol* 1994;21:207-16.

[59] O'Connell DM, Fagan WA, Skinner SM, et al. Cutaneous involvement in chronic myelomonocytic leukaemia. *Int J Dermatol* 1994;33:628-31.

[60] Schadendorf D, Algermissen B, Harmann K et al. Acute monoblastic leukemia with skin nodules in an adult. *J Am Acad Dermatol* 1993;28:884-8.

[61] Ochonisky S, Aractingi S, Dombret H, et al. Acute undifferentiated myeloblastic leukemia revealed by specific hemorrhagic bullous lesions. *Arch Dermatol* 1993;129:1301-6.

[62] Brownstein MH, Helwing EB. Patterns of cutaneous metastasis. Arch Dermatol 1972; 105: 862–68.

[63] Cohen I, Levy E, Schreiber H. Alopecia neoplastica due to breast carcinoma. *Arch Dermatol* 1961;84:490-2.

[64] Carson HJ, Pelletiere EV, Lack E. Alopecia neoplastica simulating alopecia areata and antedating the detection of primary breast carcinoma. *J Cutan Pathol* 1994;21:67-70.

[65] Mallon E, Dawber RPR. Alopecia neoplastica without alopecia: a unique presentation of breast carcinoma scalp metastasis. *J Am Acad Dermatol* 1994;31:319-21.

[66] Chen P, Middlebrook MR, Goldman SM, Sandler CM. Sister Mary Joseph nodule from metastatic renal cell carcinoma. *J Comput Assist Tompgr* 1998;22:756

[67] Sina B and Deng A. Umbilical metastasis from prostate carcinoma (Sister Mary Joseph's nodule): case report and review of literature. *J Cutan Pathol* 2007;34:581-83.

[68] Dubreuil A, Compmartin A, Barjot P, Louvet S, Leroy D. Umbilical metastasis of Sister Mary Joseph's nodule. *Int J Dermatol* 1998;37:7.

[69] Chakraborty AK, Reddy AN, Grosberg SJ, et al. Pancreatic carcinoma with dissemination to the umbilicus and skin. *Arch Dermatol* 1977;113:838-9.

[70] Chatterjee SN, Bauer HM. Umbilical metastasis from carcinoma of the pancreas. *Arch Dermatol* 1980;116;954-5.

[71] Schwartz RA, Fleishman JS. Transitional cell carcinoma of the urinary tract presenting with a cutaneous metastasis. Arch Dermatol 1981;117:513-5.

[72] Ando K-I, Goto Y, Kato K, et al. Zosteriform inflammatory metastatic carcinoma from transitional cell carcinoma of the renal pelvis. *J Am Acad Dermatol* 1994;31:284-6.

[73] Langlois NEI, McClinton S, Miller ID. An unusual presentation of transitional cell carcinoma of the distal urethra. *Histopathol* 1992;21:482-4.

[74] Schwartz RA, Rubenstein DJ, Raventos A, et al. Inflammatory metastatic carcinoma of the parotid. *Arch Dermatol* 1984;120:796-7.

[75] Faust HB, Treadwell PA. Metastatic adenocarcinoma of the scalp mimicking a kerion. *J Am Acad Dermatol* 1993;29:654-5.

[76] Jones C, Rosen T. Multiple red nodules on lower abdomen. *Arch Dermatol* 1992;128:1535-8.

[77] Venable DD, Hastings D, Misra RP. Unusual metastatic patterns of prostate adenocarcinoma. J Urol 1983;130:980-5.

[78] Andrews GC. Carcinoma of the prostate with zosteriform cutaneous lesions. *Arch Dermatol* 1971;104:301-3.

[79] Peison B. Metastasis of carcinoma of the prostate to the scalp: simulation of a large sebaceous cyst. *Arch Dermatol* 1971;104:301-3.

[80] Reingold IM, Smith BR. Cutaneous metastases from hepatomas. *Arch Dermatol* 1978;114(7):1045–6.

[81] Kubota Y, Koga T, Nakayama J. Cutaneous metastasis from hepatocellular carcinoma resembling pyogenic granuloma. *Clin Exp Dermatol* 1999;24(2):78–80.

[82] Garcia-Patos V, Castells L, Vidal J, Vargas V, De Torres I, Castells A. Cutaneous angiomatous metastasis of hepatocarcinoma. *Gastroenterol Hepatol* 1996;19(3):183–4.

[83] Yeung SN, Blicker JA, Buffam FV, et al. Metastatic eyelid disease associated with hepatocellular carcinoma. *Can J Ophthalmol* 2007;42:752-4.

[84] Youngberg GA, Berro J, Young M, et al. Metastatic epidermotropic squamous cell carcinoma histologically simulating primary carcinoma. *Am J Dermatopathol* 1989;11:457-65.

[85] Nonomura A, Shintani T, Kono N, et al. Primari carcinoid tumor of the larynx and review of the literature. *Acta Pathol Jpn* 1983;33:1041-9.

[86] Robey EL, Schellhammer PF. Four cases of metastases to the penis and a review of the literature. *J Urol* 1984;132:992-4.

[87] Cohen PR. Metastatic tumors to the nail unit: subungual metastases. *Dermatol Surg* 2001;27:280-93.

[88] Arnold AC, Bullcok JD, Foos RY. Metastatic eyelid carcinoma. *Ophthalmology* 1985;92:114-9.

[89] Riley FC. Metastatic tumors to the eyelids. *Am J Ophthalmol* 1970;69:259-64.

[90] Quecedo E, Ferber I, Martínez-Escribano JA, et al. Tumoral seeding after pericardiocentesis in a patient with a pulmonary adenocarcinoma. *J Am Acad Dermatol* 1994;31:496-7.

[91] Freund H, Biran S, Laufer N, et al. Breast cancer arising in surgical scars. *J Surg Oncol* 1976;8:477-80.

[92] Grenier DJ, Kaplan RP. Occult adenocarcinoma metastatic to a skin graft donor site. *J Dermatol Surg Oncol* 1985;11:1213-6.

[93] Ueda K, Okada N, Yoshikawa K. A case of cutaneous metastasis of bile duct carcinoma. *J Am Acad Dermatol* 1991;25:848-9.

[94] Betke M, Süss R, Hohenleutner U, et al. Gastric carcinoma metastastic to the site of a congenital melanocytic nevus. *J Am Acad Dermatol* 1993;28:866-9.

[95] Hayes AG, McChesney TM. Metastatic adenocarcinoma of the breast located within a benign intradermal nevus. Am J Dermatopathol 1993;15:280-2.

[96] Resnik KS, DiLeonardo M, Gibbons G. Clinically occult cutaneous metastases. *J Am Acad Dermatol* 2006;55:1044-7.

In: Handbook of Skin Care in Cancer Patients   ISBN: 978-1-61668-419-8
Editors: Pierre Vereecken and Ahmad Awada   © 2012 Nova Science Publishers, Inc.

Chapter 10

COSMETIC AND MEDICINAL PRODUCTS: A DISTINCT BUT COMPLEMENTARY APPROACH...?

Alain Lechien

Lecturer at the Institute of Pharmacy, Université Libre de Bruxelles, Belgium

ABSTRACT

Differentiating a cosmetic product from a medicinal product is not always easy, especially as there are many misconceptions on the subject. This article defines cosmetic and medicinal products within a European context both in relation to each other and in relation to biocidal products and medical devices. The significance of cosmetic products is also examined.

INTRODUCTION

What is a cosmetic product? This may seem like a relatively simple question... but there are several possible answers.

From a **chemical** point of view, a cosmetic product is generally a mix of hydrophilic substances, lipophilic substances and emulsifying agents to which colorants, preservatives, sun screens, etc... are added.

These substances constitute a mixture known as an "emulsion" and can either be a *O/W* emulsion if the majority part is aqueous (giving a light texture) or *W/O* if the majority part is lipophilic (giving a richer texture). Triple emulsions are also possible (*W/O/W*)...

From a **physical** point of view, a cosmetic can be either a fluid product with monophasic solution (make-up remover for the eyes, lotions, shampoos) or biphasic (such as suspension substances, emulsions, aerosols, etc) or a solid product (in the case of make-up powders or lipstick, etc...).

These characteristics do not therefore permit us to differentiate cosmetic products from medicinal products.

In reality, it is the ***legal*** viewpoint and resulting definitions which enable the distinction to be made. This legal framework is also very important because this determines the advertising claims permitted for the products as well as any possible commercial promotions.

It therefore quickly becomes clear that this legal framework is of great importance to manufacturers.

THE LEGAL FRAMEWORK

In general, a product is classed as a "*cosmetic product*" if it meets 2 conditions at the same time:

1. It *must meet* the legal definition of the cosmetic product...
2. ...and *must not meet* the legal definition of a medicinal product, biocidal product or medical device.

Such a legal framework would be ideal if it was specific about each of the categories...

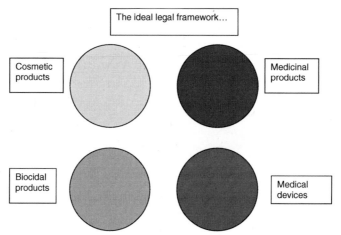

In practice, this is not the case, given the existence of "overlap" zones. . . .

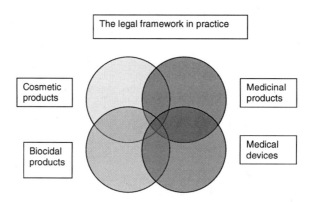

This results in a degree of legal uncertainty for products which fall in these overlap zones, known hereinafter as "border line" products.... .

LEGISLATION FOR COSMETIC PRODUCTS

In the majority of European countries, the existing (2010) cosmetic products legislation is the result of the European Directive 76/768/CEE (combined, in some countries, with specific rules).

In Belgium, the legislation specifies *3 essential preconditions* for marketing cosmetic products:

- possession of a *complete file* on the product which must be made available to the authorities: this file should contain the product's composition, raw material specifications, manufacture process, safety assessment, proof of stated effect, etc…;
- a *notification* of the products (information of the authorities-specific);
- transmission of the formulas to the Anti-Poisons Centre (specific).

Annex 1 of the directive contains a classification of cosmetic products:

Illustrative List by Category of Cosmetic Products

- Creams, emulsions, lotions, gels and oils for the skin (hands, face, feet, etc.).
- Face masks (with the exception of peeling products).
- Tinted bases (liquids, pastes, powders).
- Make-up powders, after-bath powders, hygienic powders, etc.
- Toilet soaps, deodorant soaps, etc.
- Perfumes, toilet waters and eau de Cologne.
- Bath and shower preparations (salts, foams, oils, gels, etc.).
- Depilatories.
- Deodorants and anti-perspirants.
- Hair care products:
- hair tints and bleaches,
- products for waving, straightening and fixing,
- setting products,
- cleansing products (lotions, powders, shampoos),
- conditioning products (lotions, creams, oils),
- hairdressing products (lotions, lacquers, brilliantines).
- Shaving products (creams, foams, lotions, etc.).
- Products for making up and removing make-up from the face and the eyes.
- Products intended for application to the lips.
- Products for care of the teeth and the mouth.
- Products for nail care and make-up.
- Products for external intimate hygiene.
- Sunbathing products.

- Products for tanning without sun.
- Skin-whitening products.
- Anti-wrinkle products.

This Directive also includes, for certain constituents, *negative* lists (annex 2), *restrictive* lists (annex 3) and *positive* lists (annexes 4, 6 and 7) as follows:

- annex 2 specifies the *non-permitted* constituents for cosmetic products (actually more than 1400 !);
- annex 3 specifies constituents *not permitted outside of certain conditions* (e.g. the concentration);
- annex 4 specifies the *only authorised colorants;*
- annex 6 specifies the *only authorised preservatives*;
- annex 7 specifies les *only authorised sunscreens.*

The Directive also specifies the *information which must be featured* on the product: the name of the manufacturer, product lifespan if less than 30 months; if more than 30 months, the period of validity after opening; any particular instructions for use, the function of the product and full labelling, i.e. a list of all the ingredients in order, starting with the greatest.

One article of the Directive states that a cosmetic product may not cause damage to human health:

A cosmetic product put on the market within the Community must not cause damage to human health when applied under normal or reasonably foreseeable conditions of use, taking account, in particular, of the product's presentation, its labelling, any instructions for its use and disposal as well as any other indication or information provided by the manufacturer or his authorized agent or by any other person responsible for placing the product on the Community market.

As regards the *definition* of a cosmetic product :

A "cosmetic product" shall mean any substance or preparation intended to be placed in contact with the various external parts of the human body (epidermis, hair system, nails, lips and external genital organs) or with the teeth and the mucous membranes of the oral cavity with a view exclusively or mainly to cleaning them, perfuming them, changing their appearance and/or correcting body odours and/or protecting them or keeping them in good condition.

Upon reading this definition, it is clear that *2 conditions* must be met in order to fulfil the definition of a cosmetic product:

- the place of **application**: *...to be placed in contact with the various external parts of the human body...*
- the **intended goal**: *...with a view exclusively or mainly to cleaning them,...*

By contrast, the definition does not specify any precisions or restrictions regarding the place of *action* or *mode of action* of the cosmetic product.

A) Where the place of *action* is concerned: contrary to what many believe, a cosmetic product can have an effect upon the epidermis, dermis or hypodermis!

In fact, the definition specifies the place of *application* of the product but not the place of *action*.

Some examples illustrate this fact:

    a) *anti-wrinkle and anti-stretch mark products*: wrinkles and stretch marks originate in the dermis. Products claiming an "anti-wrinkle" or "anti-stretch mark" effect should at least penetrate through to where these effects begin, i.e. the dermis.

    b) *Slimming creams*: cellulite is located in the hypodermis. The same reasoning as for the anti-wrinkle products can therefore be applied here.

    This penetrating effect has been confirmed using a very simple method. All "anti-cellulite" products contain caffeine due to its lipolytic properties. Tests were therefore carried out to measure the caffeine present in the blood of women using a slimming cream. The equivalent of ¼ of the quantity of caffeine found in a cup of coffee was found!

    This has 2 clear consequences:

    -Cosmetic products do penetrate through to the circulation system;

    -Women sensitive to caffeine should not use slimming creams *in the evening* or they will have trouble sleeping!

    c) Finally, if this is not sufficient, it should be remembered that all molecules applied to the skin are capable of penetrating the body to a certain extent (depending on the size of the molecule, physio-chemical characteristics, etc…) in accordance with Fick's laws of diffusion. It is utopian to think that a molecule will penetrate as far as the border between the dermis and epidermis and stop there!

A cosmetic product can, therefore, legally penetrate into the body through the skin – and in all likelihood it will…

The cosmetic industry also offers products which penetrate the skin to different degrees:

• *products where skin penetration has been researched*: slimming creams, anti-wrinkle and anti- stretch mark products, etc…

• *products with very low skin penetration*: make-up products *(otherwise they would serve no purpose!),* sunscreens *(they have to stay on the surface to enable protection of the layers beneath, otherwise they would be useless),* shampoos *(their role is to clean hair and not to let products into the body).*

Based on these considerations, it is logical to say that the place of *action* does not affect the definition of the cosmetic product.

A note about the "*intended goal*" featured in the definition: it states "*with a view exclusively or mainly…*"

The use of the word *"mainly"* signifies that a secondary activity (other than "cosmetic") is permitted for cosmetic products. The uncertainty continues, however, as this activity has never been specified or limited.

B) Where the *mode of action* is concerned: the mode of action for most cosmetic products is already well known. This is the case for deodorants, slimming products, "anti-hair loss" products, anti-wrinkle product, sun products, etc...For example:

- *deodorants* according generally to one of the following modes of action:
  - *anti-bacterial agents* prevent the development of bacteria on the skin which are responsible for transforming odourless sweat into a bad smell;
  - *anti-perspirants* which reduce the diameter of the sudoriferous ducts, therefore restricting the quantity of sweat released;
  - *odour absorbers* which trap the molecules responsible for the bad odour before they reach out nasal passages.
- the lipolytic properties of caffeine are the result of caffeine inhibiting phosphodiesterase, the enzyme which stops lipolysis by deactivating AMPc;
- certain "anti-wrinkle" products act by inhibiting the contraction of fibroblasts responsible for the appearance of wrinkles;
- certain "anti-hair loss" products inhibit the synthesis of lysylhydroxy-lase, the enzyme responsible for perifollicular fibrosis.

For more details, please refer to specialist literature in this field.

It is therefore logical that, here too, the mode of action of a cosmetic product, whether it can be identified with precision or is not known, does not affect the definition of a cosmetic product. Knowing or not knowing the mode of action does not determine the legal status.

To summarise, *the following cannot be considered as cosmetic products:*

1) Products which do not meet the definition of a cosmetic products where the place of *application* and *intended goal* are concerned;
2) Substances containing substances *not permitted according to annex 2* of the 76/768/CEE directive (e.g. *androgens, oestrogens, alkaloids, lidocaine, retinoic acid, minoxidil, coal tar, etc...*);
3) Products containing substances listed in *annex 3 outside of the specified conditions* (e.g. *fluoride toothpaste with more than 150 mg % of fluoride*);
4) Products containing substances *not specified in annex 4 (for colorants), 6 (for preservatives)* and *7 (for sunscreens)*;
5) Products which meet the definition of a medicinal product, biocidal substance or medical device (cf. below).

A contrario, to be considered as a cosmetic product, a product must meet the following 4 criteria at once:

- The place of application
- The intended goal   in accordance with the 76/768/CEE
- The composition
- The presentation = the claims: cannot fall within the definitions
        of a medicinal product, biocidal agent or medical device.

LEGISLATION FOR MEDICINAL PRODUCTS

The definition of a medicinal product is also specified by a European Directive (actually Directive 2004/27/CE):

Medicinal Product

(a) Any substance or combination of substances presented as having properties for treating or preventing disease in human beings;

or

(b) any substance or combination of substances which may be used in or administered to human beings either with a view to restoring, correcting or modifying physiological functions by exerting a pharmacological, immunological or metabolic action, or to making a medical diagnosis.

It should be noted that, in the 1960s, the majority of national definitions only covered the first part of the definition... but following the launch and development of the contraceptive pill, the authorities were obliged to add the 2nd part of the definition, otherwise the contraceptive pill would not have been classed as a medicinal product (pregnancy is not an "illness"!!), with all the consequences this would have created...

A product is therefore classed as a medicinal product according to:

- its *function* (preventative or curative with regard to illness, active with regard to psychological functions);
- its medicinal *presentation (galenic form, packaging, dosage, instructions for use, Latin or scientific names, presentation in foreign countries, etc...);*
- and finally by its *composition* (presence of components featuring for example in the cosmetic products directive in annex II or annex III outside of the specified conditions)

It should be noted that a product can be defined as a medicinal product independently of whether or not it possesses curative or preventative properties... the problem is not one of misleading adverts but relates to claims about such activities.

With this in mind, we should not assume something about the definition which it does not in fact say!

Take the example of a product X, with the following information featured on its packaging:

X....: covers large or localised skin blemishes perfectly.

Indications: vitiligo, angioma, couperosis, rosacea, acne, blemishes,
pigment disorders, scars, burns…

Many people would tend to assume this is a medicinal product, based on the names of the illnesses quoted (vitiligo, angioma, couperosis, rosacea, acne). However, this alone is not sufficient as, in the present case, no treatment claim is made! It is presented with purely cosmetic claims ("covers perfectly") and this product is therefore a cosmetic product.

On the other hand, it is clear that the cosmetic industry tries to avoid its products being classed as medicinal products, where possible in order to avoid:

- submission of a large registration file in advance,
- important deadlines set by the authorities to examine the product,
- delivery, by default, subject to a medical prescription,
- controls over pricing and price increases,
- all forms of advertising submitted to the authorities in advance.

These restrictions are completely useless and superfluous in the case of cosmetic products especially as, in addition to these checks, the related deadlines are inordinately disadvantageous.

In addition to legislation for medicinal products, it should also be noted that 2 other forms of legislation can affect legislation for cosmetic products, though to a lesser extent: legislation for *biocidal products* and legislation for *medical devices*.

LEGISLATION FOR BIOCIDAL PRODUCTS

The definition of biocidal products is also specified by a European directive (actually Directive 98/8/CEE)

Biocidal Products

Active substances and preparations containing one or more active substances, put up in the form in which they are supplied to the user, intended to destroy, deter, render harmless, prevent the action of, or otherwise exert a controlling effect on any harmful organism by chemical or biological means.

An exhaustive list of 23 product types with an indicative set of descriptions within each type is given in Annex V.

Annex V covers disinfectants used for human hygiene and certain other anti-parasitic products such as anti-lice products and insecticides. Certain cosmetic products may be affected by the presence of such ingredients.

LEGISLATION FOR MEDICAL DEVICES

The definition of medical devices is also specified by a European directive (actually Directive 93/42/CEE)

Medical device means any instrument, apparatus, appliance, material or other article, whether used alone or in combination, including the software necessary for its proper application intended by the manufacturer to be used for human beings for the purpose of:

- *diagnosis, prevention, monitoring, treatment or alleviation of disease,*
- *diagnosis, monitoring, treatment, alleviation of or compensation for an injury or handicap,*
- *investigation, replacement or modification of the anatomy or of a physiological process,*
- *control of conception,*

and which does not achieve its principal intended action in or on the human body by pharmacological, immunological or metabolic means, but which may be assisted in its function by such means;

Depending on the country, it is left to various different services to check adherence to this legislation. In Belgium, the situation is as follows:

- *The AFMPS (Federal Agency for Medicinal and Health Products)* deals with:
  - sterile medical materials (dressings, compresses, etc)
  - sterile materials relating to injections, perfusions, drainage and catheters
  - implants
  - devices for controlling conception and preventing STDs
  - devices which are similar to medicinal products
  - devices used in dentistry (amalgams, crowns, prosthetics)
- *The "Service Public Fédéral Economie"* (Federal Public Service Economy) deals with:
  - measuring devices, traction devices, optical devices
- *The "Agence de Contrôle Nucléaire"* (Agency for Nuclear Control) deals with:
  - PET cameras, scanners…

This discussion of cosmetic products would be incomplete without addressing the following question:

ARE COSMETIC PRODUCTS POINTLESS?

Some people would like to minimise interest in and the role played by cosmetic products. Of course, a cosmetic product cannot make claims of a therapeutic or medicinal nature. However, the following points should not be overlooked:

1) Cosmetic products are part of our everyday lives: soaps, shampoos, deodorants, make-up removers, bubble baths, lipsticks, etc.

2) Cosmetic products often constitute an *effective remedy* for the secondary effects of certain medicinal products (dry skin when using tretinoin or benzoylperoxide)

3) Cosmetic products can also provide an *alternative* to medicinal products (week 1, treatment with anti-acne product, week 2 use of a keratolytic cosmetic product)

4) Cosmetic products constitute the *only effective means of prevention* for certain pathologies: sunburn, sun allergies, sun-induced herpes, certain skin cancers, photoallergies and photoirritations, etc…

5) Certain cosmetic products are even *more effective and more pleasant* to use that their medical equivalents (certain anti-dandruff shampoos or anti-hair loss products, etc)

6) Finally, don't forget that 10% of the population suffer from severe skin complaints, that 53% of these people find it difficult to be seen by others and that one person in 3 suffers a loss of self-confidence.

The cause of this:

a) *Colour imperfections*: angiomas (8 % of the European population), vitiligo (3 % of the Caucasian population but 6% of ethnic populations), couperosis (15 % of the European population), chloasma (70 % of pregnant women); etc…

b) *Skin contour imperfections*: acne (37 % of the European population), burns (150,000 cases per year in France), scars, post-op lesions (300,000 operations in France per year: melanomas, peelings, laser, dermabrasion, etc…)

Cosmetic products are often the only alternative available for masking certain skin disorders: *vitiligo, angioma, couperosis, chloasma, rosacea, acne, blemishes, pigment disorders, scars, burns, oily skin (seborrheic dermatitis with dilated pores), dry skin (xerosis with scaly skin…)*

The use of colour correctors (containing 25 to 40% pigments) provides a highly effective means of concealing such skin complaints and many dermatology services have now developed their services with this in mind.

CONCLUSION

While there may be an obvious means of differentiating between medicinal and cosmetic products in most cases, for certain products the distinction is less evident.

A cosmetic product is characterised by: the place of *application* of the product, the *intended goal*, the fact that it should *not be harmful*.

By contrast, neither the place of *action* nor the *mode of action* have any effect on the definition!

Finally, while the world "cosmetic" is often seen to be synonymous with "superficial", this is accurate where the place of *application* is concerned, but not necessarily where the place of action, mode of action or psychological consequences for the user are concerned :cosmetic products often constitute the only means of concealing certain skin defects… !

April 2010

REFERENCES

"Cosmetic products" directive: http://ec.europa.eu/enterprise/cosmetics

"Medicinal products" directive:
http://ec.europa.eu/enterprise/pharmaceuticals

"Biocidal products" directive:
http://ec.europa.eu/enterprise/sectors/medical-devices/other-related-policies/index_en.htm

"Medical devices" directive:
http://ec.europa.eu/enterprise/medical_devices/legislation_en.htm

In: Handbook of Skin Care in Cancer Patients   ISBN: 978-1-61668-419-8
Editors: Pierre Vereecken and Ahmad Awada   © 2012 Nova Science Publishers, Inc.

Chapter 11

MANAGEMENT OF LOWER LIMB EDEMA IN CANCER PATIENTS

Leduc Olivier[1], Delathouwer Olivier[2], Titeca Géraldine[3], Vereecken Pierre[4] and Leduc Albert[5]

[1]Lympho-phlebology Unit, Haute Ecole P.H. Spaak, Brussels, Belgium
[2]Plastic Surgeon, Chirec, Brussels, Belgium
[3]Hôpital Notre-Dame, Gosselies, Belgium
[4]Cliniques Universitaires Saint-Luc, Brussels, Belgium
[5]Prof. Emeritus Brussels Universities, Brussels, Belgium

ABSTRACT

Lower limb edema remains the most common complication after cancer treatment that produces an obstruction of the lymphatic system resulting in a decreased draining capacity.

The authors describe briefly the physiology and physiopathology of the lymphatic system even as the etiology and the stages of the edema.

The physical treatment of the edema is described during and after the hospitalization.

Finally, the surgical treatment of the edema is also evoked.

INTRODUCTION

Lymphedema of the lower extremity is a condition of localized protein-rich fluid retention in the interstitial spaces caused by a compromised lymphatic system and resulting in an abnormal enlargement of the affected part. This affection seems quite frequent in cancer patients and in this article the authors will review its causes and consequences.

PHYSIOLOGY OF THE LYMPHATIC SYSTEM

The lymphatic system is composed of thin lined-channels that transport fluid, proteins and particles that have escaped from the intravascular system to the interstitial compartment (fig. 1).

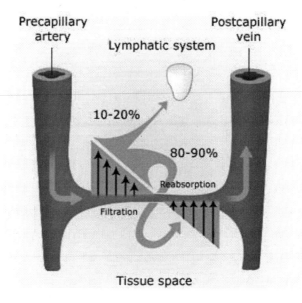

Figure 1. Filtration and reabsorption of fluid on the blood capillary level.

This fluid quit the interstitial compartment by the most distal initial lymphatics (lymph capillaries) and is then driven successively to lymph precollectors, lymph collectors and finally lymph trunks that empty in some major central veins to bring it back to the vascular system. In addition to these channels there exist lymph nodes between lymph collectors and lymph trunks. These bean-shaped encapsulated lymphatic organs have a complex function. Among others, there exists a *protective* function that results from there filter-like action for harmful elements existing in the lymph (e.g. cancer cells, bacteria,...). These elements are presented to the immune system resulting in direct and indirect immune responses.

The amount of fluid and proteins that goes out of the vascular system to the interstitial space (= the lymphatic load) and that is reabsorbed by the lymphatic system depends from several factors. In the physiologic state there is an adjusted balance between the lymphatic load and the reabsorbtion and there is no accumulation of fluid in the interstitial space. There exists a functional reserve of reabsorbtion by the lymphatic system, meaning that the reabsorption capacity can increase several-fold if the lymphatic load increases.

PHYSIOPATHOLOGY

Once that the bases of the physiology are known, it is easy to understand that any cause resulting in a decrease of the reabsorption capacity of the lymphatic system or in an increase of the lymphatic load (increased blood capillary filtration or decreased venous reabsorption) can result in an unbalanced situation. If the functional reserve of reabsorption is passed over, fluid accumulates in the interstitial space. In lymphedema, this fluid is particularly rich in proteins (1-5gm/dl) whereas protein in venous edema fluid is below 1gm/dl.

LYMPHOEDEMA STAGING

Regardless of its ethiology, lymphedema is a progressive condition that, if lefted untreated, will gradually progress through different stages (table 1)

Table 1   edema staging
Stage 0   Subclinical state: swelling is not evident despite impaired lymph   transport
Stage I   Represents early onset of the condition where there is accumulation of tissue fluid that subsides with limb elevation. Oedema may be pitting.
Stage II   Limb elevation rarely reduces swelling and pitting is manifest
Stage III Tissue is hard (fibrotic) and no pitting. Skin changes such as thickening, hyperpigmentation, increased skin folds, fat deposits warty overgrowths develop

There also exists a classification of severity that results from volume comparison between the affected and the unaffected sides. Lymphedema is considered as *mild* when the volume excess of the affected limb is less than 20 % compared to the opposite side, as *moderate* if the excess is between 20 and 40 % and *severe* when the excess is more than 40 %.

The classification will also take into account other factors as *the Stemmer sign* that describes the presence of a thickened skin fold at the base of the second toe that is a diagnostic sign for lymphedema. A positive Stemmer sign occurs when this tissue cannot be lifted but can only be grasped as a lump of tissue. In a negative result, it is possible to lift the tissue normally. The state of subcutaneous tissue where local pressure produces pitting (positive) or not (negative),presence of cellulit*is* aspect of the skin or of erysipelas. Finally, the classification may also take into account the physical and psychosocial impact of the lymphedema.

CAUSES OF LYMPHEDEMA

There exist a lot of causes that can result in lymphedema.

Secondary lymphoedema, after cancer treatment, is more frequent and results from different acquired causes that produce either an obstruction of the lymphatic system resulting in a decreased reabsorption capacity. The most common cause of lower limb lymphedema is cancer and its treatment is surgery but also radiation therapy. A synergistic effect can results from association of several causes including recurrent lymphangitis, trauma, immobility, extrinsic compression due to nonmalignant states, venous disease, chronic wounds, severe obesity, …

QUALITY OF LIFE

Few studies have evaluated lymphedema after gynecological cancer treatment.

Beesley et al. [2] publish that after gynecological cancer treatment diagnosed lymphedema was more prevalent (36 %) amongst vulvar cancer treatment. The gynecological cancer survivers have higher supportive care needs in the information and symptom management domains compared with those who have no edema.

Disease severity and early onset lymphedema are associated with a decreased quality of life. Limitation of physical activities is one of the most distressing aspects of lymphedema.

Muscle weakness and sensory impairment both contribute to accentuate a progressive deterioration in the patient's quality of life and body image.

The quality of life is significantly reduced in both physical and mental health as well as social interaction [3].

LYMPHEDEMA RELATED TO CANCER

Cancer evolution and oncological surgery is the leading cause of lymphedema of the lower limb.

Concerning cancer evolution, different factors can be responsible for lymphedema formation. It can result from the local growth of any primary cancer in the neighborhood of the lymphatic way. First, obstruction will result from an extrinsic mechanical compression and second, from an infiltration of the lymphatic structures blocking the flow of lymph. Of course, primary lymphatic neoplasias (lymphomas) that grow directly inside the lymphatic system will be responsible for its direct obstruction. In addition to the local growth of a primary tumor, some cancers are able to spread metastasis either by the bloodstream or by the lymphatics, developing secondary tumors in the lymph vessels or in the lymph nodes that can also compress or obstruct the lymphatics. However lymphatic metastasis can results from any neoplasm, carcinomas (cancers from epithelial origin) are more lymphophilic (testicular carcinomas, melanomas,…).

POSTSURGICAL LYMPHEDEMA

As the lymph nodes, laid on the dissemination pathway of tumour cells, form preferred receptacles, cancer surgery does not only remove tumours but also the lymph nodes.

Lymph node dissection of the groin is the most common cause of acquired lymphedema of the lower limbs in developed countries. Anatomically the groin includes inguinal nodes that are superficial (nodes superficial to the abdominal wall and nodes from the femoral triangle) and pelvic nodes that are deep (iliac and obturator nodes). Literature gives incidence of lymphedema after groin dissection that ranges from 20% [4,5] to 64% [6]. As suggested by Bergmark [7] it is reasonable to estimate that lymphedema incidence is surgery dependent, varying with the surgical technique and with the extend of the lymphadenectomy.

In addition to that there is an absence of consensus regarding the definition of lymphedema used in the follow-up of the patients in different series. However, for melanomas [8] as for penile carcinomas [5] or gynecologic cancers [7,8,10] the incidence increases with the extension of the dissection, deep (ilioinguinal) dissection resulting in more lymhedema than superficial dissection. All authors agree too to say that the proportion of female patients who developed lymphedema after gynaecological cancer surgery is statistically larger in cases of pelvic lymph node removal with concurrent radiotherapy. The type of incision has its importance too, S-shaped incisions resulting more often in lymphatic collection and stagnation, with a higher incidence of wound infections and leg edema than straight incisions [11].

Under optimal healing conditions, transected lymphatic ducts are able to regenerate and to reestablish a lympho-lymphatic anastomose between proximal and distal stumps across a gap of approximately 1 mm. The distal end of a severed lymph collector may also connect with an adjacent vein by a lympho-venous anastomosis, creating a natural shunt were lymph fluid goes directly in the venous blood [12]. Any concomitant process resulting in increased fibrosis of the operative field may hindered this regenerative process contributing to a higher risk of lymphedema. Among these processes, we can quote radiation therapy, postoperative infection [4,13], delayed healing and all the other causes of secondary lymphedema.

In the management of early stage melanomas, development of the sentinel lymph node (SLN) biopsy by Morton in the 1990 [14] dramatically reduced the indications for elective lymph nodes dissections (ELND). Because the SLN is the first nodal drainage site of the tumor, its tumor status can be used to predict the tumor status of all nodes in the regional basin. ELND will be proposed only to the patient with tumor involved SLN. Although complications following SLN biopsy is lower than after ELND, some series report lymphedema incidence of 0,6 [15] to 6% [6]. Beyond its wide acceptance in melanoma and breast cancer management, SLN biopsy is increasingly indicated in other cancers as sarcomas [15,16], vulvar cancers [17], penile cancers [18], mucous or skin squamous cell carcinomas [19] … .

Management of Lymphedema

The Lymphatic Pathways of Vicariousness

On a vascular point of view it is well known that the blood flow interruption can subside with the elaboration of a collateral circulation. We did proof the existence of similar abilities in the lymphatic circulation. In that regard, collateral pathways were first put forward in an animal study (Leduc A, Lievens P) [20] and subsequently in human dissections (Leduc A, Caplan I, Leduc O) [21]. We have visualized these lymphatic pathways on the upper as well as on the lower limbs(Figure 2a,b).

In a subsequent study the same pathways were observed from cancer surgical patients who did receive the physical treatment recommended by the consensus [22] (Figure 3.a,b).

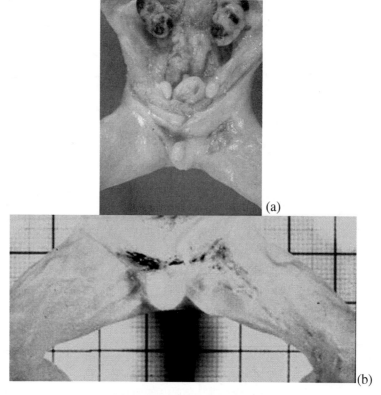

Figure 2 (a) and (b). Inguino-inguinal pathways after left limb Gerota mass injection.

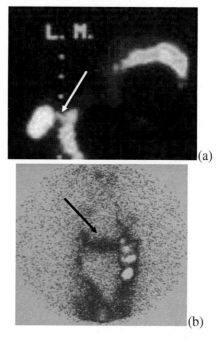

Figure 3 (a) and (b). Inguino-inguinal pathways by patient. Visualisation by mean of lymphoscinti-graphy. (P. Bourgeois).

The physical treatment (see below) seems to be preponderant.
The rehabilitation of the patient is divided as follows:

i.   *inpatient treatment*
ii.   *post-hospitalization outpatient*
iii. *long-term treatment*
iv.   *treatment during radiotherapy or chemotherapy*

L.M. = midline; arrow indicates the inguino-inguinal pathways.

Rehabilitation during Hospitalization

a.   *Treatment when there is no edema* depending of the surgical approach
      The re-education of the mobility is ongoing.
      The preventive measures and care of the limb are gradually introduced.
      Manual lymphatic drainage is already recommend if the patient feels a sensation of swelling.
b. *treatment with existing edema*
      The edema may appear during hospitalisation but, at this stage, it is still minimal [26].
      Treatment is identical but the physiotherapist also carries out daily manual lymphatic drainage.
      Note: during hospitalization, excess mobilisation may induce "lymph" which in itself can induce a "lymphocele" or seroma.

Post Hospitalization Outpatient
      Lower limb edema, post cancer surgery generally appears during the first year [26]. Commonly recognised situations are:

a.   *Edema not present:* Treatment is not necessary but preventive measures must be recognised by the patient.
b.   *Slight edema:* size of the edema is less than 20% compared to the healthy side. Manual lymphatic drainage is recommended 3 to 5 times per week for 2 or3 weeks, followed by reducing sessions until the end of the treatment.
c.   *The edema is moderate or severe:* the size of the edema is more than 20% compared to the healthy side. The edema will be treated according to of the International Society of Lymphology consensus document [22].

First Stage: Intensive Care
      Manual lymphatic drainage (MLD)
      Low pressure intermittent pneumatic compression pressotherapy (IPC).
      Multilayer bandages.
      Treatment frequency: 5 times per week during 2 to 3 weeks [23]
      Duration: ½ hour for MLD, 1 hour for low pressure IPC (with a pressure of 20 to 40 mm Hg)

Application of the multilayer bandaging that must be worn day and night.

The patient remains active and proceeds with normal activities of daily living.

Sport activities are not advisable at this stage.

Second Stage of Treatment

Manual lymphatic drainage (MLD)

Low pressure intermittent pneumatic compression therapy

Compression hosiery

Treatment frequency: 5, 3 and eventually weekly

Duration: ½ hour for the manual lymphatic drainage and 1 hour for IPC

The treatment is initially commenced daily for 2-3 weeks and depending on clinical results the frequency is progressively reduced to eventually once a week.

Some patients will require long term ongoing weekly MLD, others will not.

The total duration of treatment depends of the severity of the edema and its stabilisation.

Initially, compression garments should be worn 24 hours per day.

Once maintained this can be reduced to daytime only and depending on progress and maintenance, the therapist may be able to reduce the wear of the compression garments.

Long Term Treatment

Some resistant, chronic edemas will require long term regular treatment.

This treatment requires regular manual lymphatic drainage, usually weekly.

The therapist will instruct the patient on appropriate physical activities and exercise in order to improve her/his quality of life [27]. Some sport activities are not advisable [24, 25].

Wearing compression hosiery is helpful and often essential according to the etiology of the oedema. If venous sufficiency is compromised it is essential to wear compression garments. However if only lymphatic insufficiency is present the patient can gradually reduce the wear of the stocking and eventually stop.

It is recommended that all patients should wear compression for long journeys by car or train or when flying.

Surgical Treatment

Although the cornerstone of treatment for patient with lymphedema involves compression garment use as well as multilayers bandaging and lymphatic massage, some patients are unresponsive to conservative therapy. For these patient different surgical therapies have been proposed. Procedures are traditionally divided into physiologic procedures that attempt to restore normal drainage patterns and excisional procedures that remove lymphedematous tissue. Physiologic procedures include lymphangio-plasties, buried dermal flaps, omental transpoisions, lymph node-venous anastomosis, microlymphaticovenous anastomosis and microsurgical lymphatic grafting among others. Excisional procedures include radical excision, staged subcutaneous excisions or liposuction as promoted by Brorson [28]. It is very important to note that none of these surgical procedures have reproducible, proven efficacity in reversing the physiopathology of the lymphedematous process. Even though there seems to be a noticeable enhancement in the clinical status of the patients presented in the major part of these series, it is impossible to attest that this enhancement results from the surgical procedure and not from the intensive physical therapy that systematically accompanies the postoperative period.

Skin Care

Skin care is also of the utmost importance. Water soluble ointments as emollients, with 2 to 5 percent salicylic acid can prevent or treat excessive hyperkeratosis. Regular washing followed by antiseptic drying agent is essential to avoid bacteria flourish in deep crevices. Control of bacterial or fungal infection is essential. Eczema can often both contribute to and result from lymphoedema and may require transient topical steroids. A less frequent but more severe complication of such a chronic lymphedema is the "Stewart-Treves syndrome" consisting in a 3-year-median survival lymphangiosarcoma and presenting clinically as violaceous cutaneous papules and plaques surrounding the lymphedema.

REFERENCES

[1] The diagnosis and treatment of peripheral lymphedema.Consensus of the Executive. Commity. *Lymphology* 2003; 36 (2): 84-91.

[2] Beesley V, Janda M, Eakin E, Obermair A, Battittusta D Lymphedema after gynecological cancer treatment: prevalence, correlates, and supportive care needs. *Cancer,*2007 Jun 15; 109(12):2607-14.

[3] Pereira DE Godoy JM, Bralle DM, de Fatima Godoy M, Longo O Jr : Quality of life and peripheral lymphedema. *Lymphology 2002 Jun;* 35(2):72-5.

[4] Rapaport DP, Stadelmann WK, Reintgen DS. Inguinal lymphadenectomy. In Balch CM, Houghton AN, Milton GW et al., eds. Cutaneous Melanoma, 3d ed. Philadelphia : *JB Lippincot,* 1998, p 279.

[5] Ravi R. Morbidity following groin dissection for penile carcinoma.*Br J Urol.* 1993 Dec;72(6):941-5.

[6] de Vries M, Vonkeman WG, van Ginkel RJ, Hoekstra HJ..Morbidity after inguinal sentinel lymph node biopsy and completion lymph node dissection in patients with cutaneous melanoma. *Eur J Surg Oncol.* 2006 Sep;32(7):785-9. Epub 2006 Jun 27.

[7] Bergmark K. & al. Lymphedema and bladder-emptying difficulties after radical hysterectomy for early cervical ca:413-8ncer and among population controls. *Int J Gynecol Cancer.* 2006 ; 16: 1130-1139.

[8] Beitsch P, Balch C.Operative morbidity and risk factor assessment in melanoma patients undergoing inguinal lymph node dissection. *Am J Surg.* 1992 Nov;164(5):462-5; discussion 465-6.

[9] Werngren-Elgstrom M., Lidman L. Lymphoedema of the lower extremities after surgery and radiotherapy for cancer of the cervix. *Scand J. Plast Reconstr Hand Surg.* 1994; 28: 289-293.

[10] Ryan M. Stainton MC,Jaconelli C, Mackenzie P, Mansberg T. The experience of lower limb lymphedema for woman after treatment for gynaecologic cancer. Onco; *Nurs Forum* 2003; Vol. 30 (3): 417-23.

[11] Tonouchi H, Ohmori Y, Kobayashi M, Konishi N, Tanaka K, Mohri Y, Mizutani H, Kusunoki M. Operative morbidity associated with groin dissections. *Surg Today.* 2004;34(5):413-8.

[12] Zuther JE. Lymphedema Management. *The comprehensive guide for practitioners.* Thieme Medical Publishers, 2005.

[13] James JH. Lymphoedema following ilio-inguinal lymph node dissection.*Scand J Plast Reconstr Surg.* 1982;16(2):167-71.

[14] Morton, D.; Cagle, L.; Wong, J., et al. Intraoperative lymphatic mapping and selective lymphadenectomy: technical details of a new procedure for clinical stage I melanoma. Presented at t*he Annual Meeting of the Society of Surgical Oncology;* Washington, DC. 1990.

[15] Roaten JB, Pearlman N, Gonzalez R, Gonzalez R, McCarter MD.Identifying risk factors for complications following sentinel lymph node biopsy for melanoma. *Arch Surg.* 2005 Jan;140(1):85-9.

[16] Blazer DG 3rd, Sabel MS, Sondak VK. Is there a role for sentinel lymph node biopsy in the management of sarcoma? *Surg Oncol.* 2003 Nov;12(3):201-6.

[17] Hauspy J, Beiner M, Harley I, Ehrlich L, Rasty G, Covens A Sentinel lymph node in vulvar cancer. *Cancer.* 2007 Sep 1;110(5):1015-23.

[18] Perdonà S, Autorino R, De Sio M, Di Lorenzo G, Gallo L, Damiano R, D'Armiento M, Gallo A. Dynamic sentinel node biopsy in clinically node-negative penile cancer versus radical inguinal lymphadenectomy: a comparative study. *Urology.* 2005 Dec;66(6):1282-6.

[19] Sahn RE, Lang PG. Sentinel lymph node biopsy for high-risk nonmelanoma skin cancers. *Dermatol Surg.* 2007 Jul;33(7):786-92; discussion 792-3.

[20] Leduc A., Lievens P. : Les anastomoses lympho-lymphatiques : incidences thérapeutiques. *Travaux de SSBK,* vol IV, n° 1, 1976.

[21] Leduc A., Caplan I., Leduc O. : Lymphatic drainage of the upper limb. Substitution lymphatic pathways. *Eur. J. of Lymphology and Rel. Probl.* vol. 4, n° 13, 1993.

[22] International Society of Lymp"Hology, Diagnosis and treatment of peripheral lympedema. Consenus document; *Lymphology* 2003 ;36 (2) :84-91.

[23] Leduc, O., Leduc, A., Bourgeois, P., Belgrado, J-P. The physical treatment of upper limb edema. *Cancer* 1998 ; 83 :2835-9.

[24] BOURGeOIS P, *Leduc A Lymphoscintigraphic evaluation of the lower limbs in soccers: about 6 cases Médecine Nucléaire Vol 31,* Issue 1, Jan07, pp10-15.

[25] Johansson K, Tibe k, Weibull A, Newton R.U. Low intensity resistance exercise for breast cancer patients with arm lyphedema with or without compression sleeve. *Lymphology dec* 05 Vol 38, n°4.

[26] Cohen S.R.; Payne D.K., Tunkel R.S. Lymphedema strategies for management. *Cancer,* 2001; 92(S4): 980-987.

[27] Mock V, Pickett M, Ropka ME, Lin EM, Stewart KJ :Fatigue and quality of life outcomes of exercise during cancer treatment. *Cancer Practice,* 2001 May/Jun; 9(3): 119.

[28] Brorson H, Svensson H. Complete reduction of lymphoedema of the arm by liposuction after breast cancer. *Scand J Plast Reconstr Surg Hand Surg.* 1997 Jun;31(2):137-43.

In: Handbook of Skin Care in Cancer Patients
Editors: Pierre Vereecken and Ahmad Awada

ISBN: 978-1-61668-419-8
© 2012 Nova Science Publishers, Inc.

Chapter 12

KELOIDS AND HYPERTROPHIC SCARS AFTER SURGERY IN CANCER PATIENTS

*D. Franck, A. De Mey and W. D. Boeckx**

Department Plastic Surgery, Brugmann ULB Hospital, Brussels, Belgium

ABSTRACT

After a dermal injury, the biochemical process of wound repair initiates a complex series of events that results in the deposition of a collagen-rich matrix. In certain individuals, the repair process may be pathologic and result in large, raised collagenous scars known as keloids or hypertrophic scars, both characterized by excessive collagen deposition. The two key differences between keloid and hypertrophic scar are the 'time-line' and the association with contraction. The pathogenesis of keloids is complex and involves both genetic and environmental factors. Although there is no single definitive treatment modality, there are numerous therapeutic regiments that have been described. In our own experience the application of 24 hours per day pressure therapy, especially for hypertrophic facial burns scars , during an eighteen months period, has proven to be effective and we have published the good results of brachytherapy for the treatment of keloids of variable origin. A broad revue of the literature about keloids shows that there is no publication demonstrating an increased risk to develop keloids after cancer surgery but well an increased risk of infection and wound healing delay because of the immune and nutritional status of the patient and those are two important risk factors for the development of keloid scars.

INTRODUCTION

After a dermal injury, the biochemical process of wound repair initiates a complex series of events that results in the deposition of a collagen-rich matrix. The wound healing process is divided in three distinct phases, inflammatory-proliferative-remodeling, and can take months

---

* Author for correspondence. W.D. Boeckx, MD., PhD. willy.boeckx@chu-brugmann.be

to complete. At the end of the process, although the mature scar has not the high degree of organization as the normal dermis, it has the aspect of a fine_ line.

In certain individuals, however, the repair process may be pathologic and result in large, raised collagenous scars known as keloids or hypertrophic scars. Both lesions are unique to man, can cause itching, tenderness and pain and are characterized by excessive collagen deposition.

The clinical course defines keloid and hypertrophic scar as separate entities (Table 1).

Table 1. Clinical distinction between hypertrophic and keloid scars

	Hypertrophic Scar	Keloid scar
Overall incidence	More common	Less common
Association with race	No	More common among dark pigmented ethnicities
Always preceded by injury	Yes	Yes but may be very minimal trauma, microtrauma + infection
Anatomical association	No	Areas particularly prone: earlobes, deltoid region, presternal region
Extend of growth	Confined to area of original injury	Extends to surrounding tissue
Spontaneous resolution	Mostly	No
Recurrence after surgery	No	Yes
Association with contracture	Yes	No
Elevation	Flatten spontaneously with time	> 4 mm

Normal and hypertrophic scars are similar in terms of their 'cycle' of matrix proliferation, stabilization, and maturation. Keloid scars rarely 'mature,' but there are gross morphologic differences between mild and severe keloids.

The two key differences between keloid and hypertrophic scar are the 'time-line' and the association with contraction (Figure 1). [1]

The pathogenesis of keloids is complex and involves both genetic and environmental factors. It is widely accepted that most of the keloids develop subsequent to injury or inflammation of the skin, but the exact pathogenesis is still unknown. Wound healing delay and wound infection are two important risk factors.

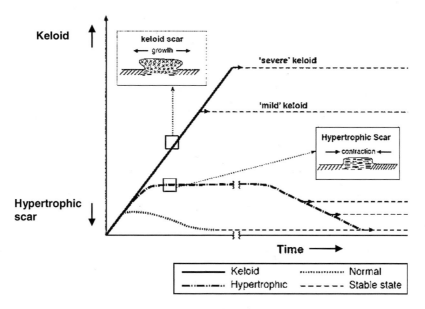

Figure 1. One essential clinical difference between hypertrophic and keloid scars is contraction of the hypertrophic scar.

KELOID AND CANCER

Keloids are benign dermal fibroproliferative tumors unique to humans with no malignant potential. Keloid scarring is a clinical diagnosis and, given a good clinical suspicion of keloid, it may be unnecessary to send specimens for routine histology [2].

Differential Diagnosis

Dermatofibrosarcoma protuberans (DFSP) [3] is a fibrohistiocytic tumor of intermediate malignancy, characterized by frequent local recurrences unless widely excised. It accounts for approximately <0.1% of all malignancies and 1% of all sarcomas. It most commonly presents in early to mid-adult life, although a wide age range may be affected. Typically, it arises as a plaque on the trunk or proximal extremities, which may subsequently develop a nodular or multinodular mass. It has a slight male preponderance. Its diagnosis is histologic, typically demonstrating slender spindle cells, radially arranged, and with a highly cellular center with tentacle-like projections at the periphery.

Keloidal basal cell carcinoma [4] is a basal cell carcinoma that presents as nodules resembling a keloid and contains keloidal collagen. It has only rarely been described. Microscopic examination demonstrated thick, sclerotic, brightly eosinophilic staining collagen bundles intermingled with characteristic basaloid epithelial aggregations of basal cell carcinoma.

Carcinoma en cuirasse is a form of metastatic cutaneous breast malignancy occurring most commonly on the chest as a recurrence of breast cancer, but it can be the primary presentation. It presents sometimes as unusual keloid-like nodules on the chest that fail to respond to therapy [5].

Non tumoral lesions: acne keloidalis, hypertrophic scar, dermatofibroma, foreign body granuloma, and the fungal infection lobomycosis.

CURRENT THERAPIES AND FUTURE PROSPECTS

Although there is no single definitive treatment modality, there are numerous therapeutic regiments that have been described, including occlusive dressings, compression therapy, intralesional steroid injections, cryosurgery, surgical excision, laser treatment, radiation therapy, interferon therapy, bleomycin, 5-fluorouracil, verapamil, imiquimod cream,TGF-β3, interleukin-10 , and combinations of all of these.

Both silicone and non-silicone–based occlusive dressings have been widely used for keloids for the last 30 years. Results from several studies have revealed 79% to 90% improvement in keloid scars with the use of these occlusive dressings, complete resolution has not been noted [6, 7].

Pressure devices or dressings have been another noninvasive treatment modality with wound improvement in 70% to 90%, but once again complete resolution has not been shown [7].

The advantage of both occlusive and pressure therapy is that although they might not completely eliminate the keloid, they tend to be better tolerated than the other more invasive therapies in pediatric patients and some adults.

Surgical excision alone has been repeatedly proven to be ineffective, with reported recurrence rates of 55% to 100% [8].The combination of surgical excision with other modalities, such as corticosteroid injection, steroid injection with pressure dressing, x-ray therapy, interstitial radiation, single fraction radiation, teletherapy radiation, and brachytherapy have revealed relatively good results, with recurrence rates reported from 8% to 72% [8, 9].

In our own experience, for hypertrophic scars, the application of 24 hours per day pressure therapy, especially for hypertrophic facial burns scars, during an eighteen months period, has proven to be effective as seen in Figure 2,3,4,5.

For keloids, various forms of radiotherapy have been attempted as a monotherapy for keloids but remain quite controversial. Radiotherapy was first introduced as a treatment in 1906 and 100 years later there is still debate about whether it is a save modality.

When used as a monotherapy, radiation is not very effective (a recurrence rate of 50–100%) [10] unless large doses are used. However, this may lead to squamous cell carcinoma of the skin of the treated sites 15 to 30 years later.

It has been shown in epidemiological studies that ionizing radiation carries a risk of carcinogenesis [11]. In particular, an increased incidence of breast cancer has been observed in women given radiotherapy for post-partum mastitis [12].

Despite the potential risks, there are very few reports in the literature of malignancies arising from the treatment of keloids with radiotherapy. The few that are reported are in patients irradiated at a young age, which appears to be the greatest risk factor [13].

Primary radiation can be very successful in alleviating the pruritus, pain and tenderness of keloids.

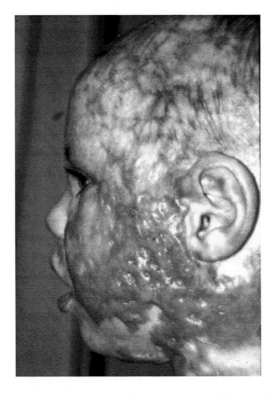

Figure 2. Hypertrophic facial burns scar after a daily treatment with Silver sulfadiazine cream in a fat fire burn.

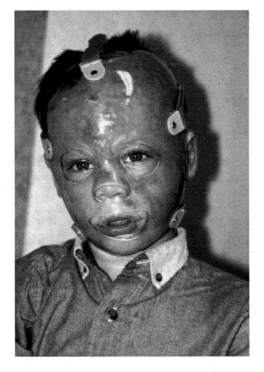

Figure 3. 24 hours daily pressure therapy with a transparent Uvex plastic face mask.

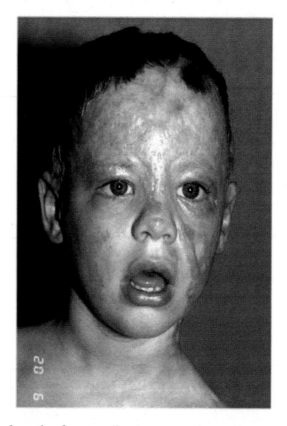

Figure 4. Situation after 6 months of pressure therapy.

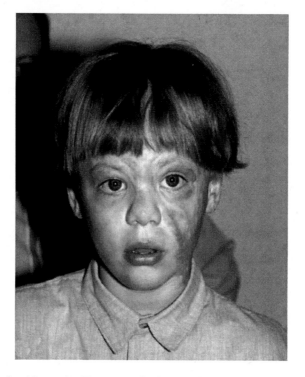

Figure 5. Final result after 18 months. Extreme softening and flattening of the hypertrophic area.

Moreover, some cases reported in the literature [13, 14] show a clear difference between the irradiated breast scar after mastectomy and the non irradiated contralateral breast symmetrisation scar. Those case reports demonstrate the effect radiotherapy had in preventing hypertrophic scars or keloid formation. Direct comparison can be made between both irradiated and non-irradiated skin within the same individual, thus eliminating many other variables.

Laser therapy using argon, CO2, and pulse dye have been attempted but none of them have proven to be efficacious. All three forms of laser therapy have recurrence rates of upwards of 90%, showing little to no benefit. [16, 17, 18, 19]

Despite pain at the therapeutic site and hypo- or hyperpigmentation, cryotherapy has proven to be quite effective as a monotherapy, with one study revealing that 73% of patients had substantial flattening of their keloid scars.[20] Additionally, of those scars that did respond, there were no recurrences reported.

Intralesional corticosteroid injections have been a relatively effective first-line therapy for the treatment of keloids. The numerous side effects: need for multiple injections, injection pain, skin atrophy, telangiectasias, and altered pigmentation have caused clinicians and researchers to continue to look for other means of treatment.

Several pharmacologic agents have recently emerged as promising treatments for keloid scars: intralesional 5-fluorouracil or bleomycin tattooing.

There are also reports of several other medications, when used in conjunction with surgical excision: postsurgical intralesional interferon injections, intralesional verapamil injections, and topical imiquimod cream.

In our own experience we have published the good results of brachytherapy for the treatment of keloids of variable origin [15] .In 24 patients 35 keloids were treated with surgical excision into healthy skin and dermis. A plastic flexible catheter (outer diameter 1.8 mm) was positioned parallel to the wound edges at a maximum depth of 5 mm. The subcutaneous tissue and skin was sutured above the catheter with an intradermal suture. The iridium 192 high-dose-rate (HDR) brachytherapy was delivered within 24 hours after surgery. With an average photon energy of 380keV, a dose of 7 Gy was delivered. The following day, another dose of 7 Gy was again delivered. Thereafter, the catheter was removed at the outpatient clinic. The long term results were evaluated in 30 keloids. There were 14 male and 10 female patients. The mean age was 41.6 years (range 22-76 years), 41.7% of patients being over the 30. Nineteen patients (79%) were Caucasian and 21% with darker skin (African, Indonesian, Indians). The time interval between the keloid growing and skin trauma was in most cases between 0 and 6 months (63%), between 6 and 12 months for 4 keloids (13%), and after 12 months for the remaining keloids (10%). The location of the keloids is given in table 2. The etiology is given in table 3 and the results in table 4. Preoperative keloid thickness and width was measured in 26 out of 30 scars. The mean thickness was 5.65 mm (range: 2-16 mm), the mean width was 17.54 mm (range: 2-50 mm) and preoperative mean length was 10.8 cm (range: 0.3 -31 cm). In 87% of patients there was no family history of keloid.

Our surgical and brachytherapy treatment was the first ever treatment in 9 patients (30%) and in 8 patients (27%) the keloids had been treated before. 13 keloids (43%) received different unsuccessful treatments before, including corticosteroid injections, Silastic sheet coverage, surgical excisions, Elastogel and Laser therapy.

The photographically recorded results were evaluated by a panel of 3 laymen, 5 professionals and all patients. The mean follow up was 27 months   (range: 8-58).

Table 2. Location of keloid scars

Location	Frequency	Percentage
Arms/Hands	3	10
Heah+Neck	8	26.7
Breast	17	56.7
Back	1	3.3
Abdomen	1	3.3
Total	30	100

Table 3. Etiology of keloid scars

Etiology	Percentage
Sternotomy	20
Breast reduction	10
Laparotomy	3.3
Otoplasty	13.4
Ear piercing	10
Shoulder operation	6.7
Small surgery	6.7
Burn injury	6.7
Acne	3.3
Insect bite	3.3
Other	16.6

Table 4. Evaluations by laymen, professionals and patients

	Laymen	Professionals	Patients
Very bad	1.1%	0%	3.3%
Bad	8.9%	0.7%	6.7%
Not so good	18.9%	13.3%	10%
Quite good	26.7%	26.7%	23.3%
Good	26.7%	38%	50%
Very good	4.4%	8%	>3.3%
Missing	13.3%	13.3%	3.3%

We observed a significant difference in scar thickness before (5.65 mm ± 3.58) and after the treatment (0.39 mm ± 0.63 mm, $p< 0.001$). Moreover, in all patients the post op thickness was less than 2 mm. There was no effect related to the anatomic location of the keloid on the body, length of keloid, patient's age, and gender or skin color. No complications occurred except for one patient with a wound infection and consequent wound breakdown, causing a 3 cm wound dehiscence, finally resulting in a spontaneous healing without keloid recurrence.

CONCLUSION

A broad revue of the literature about keloids shows that there is no publication demonstrating an increased risk to develop keloids after cancer surgery but well an increased risk after infection and wound healing delay because of the continuous local inflammatory reaction.

For the last ten years a lot of work and progress have been done about wound healing but there is still a lack of studies about keloids.

REFERENCES

[1]   Burd A, Huang L. Hypertrophic response and keloid diathesis: two very different forms of scar. *Plast Reconstr Surg* 2005;116:150e-7e.

[2]   Wong TW, Lee JY. Should excised keloid scars be sent for routine histologic analysis? *Ann Plast Surg*. 2008 Jun;60(6):724.

[3]   Yu W, Tsoukas MM, Chapman SM, Rosen JM. Surgical treatment for dermatofibrosarcoma protuberans: the Dartmouth experience and literature review. *Ann Plast Surg*. 2008 Mar;60(3):288-93.

[4]   Lewis JE. Keloidal basal cell carcinoma. *Am J Dermatopathol*. 2007 Oct;29(5):485.

[5]   Mullinax K, Cohen JB. Carcinoma en cuirasse presenting as keloids of the chest. *Dermatol Surg*. 2004 Feb;30(2 Pt 1):226-8.

[6]   Wong TW, Chiu HC, Chang CH, Lin LJ, Liu CC, Chen JS. Silicone cream occlusive dressing—a novel noninvasive regimen in the treatment of keloid. *Dermatology* 1996;192:329–333.

[7]   Bieley HC, Berman B. Effects of a water-impermeable, nonsilicone-based occlusive dressing on keloids. *J Am Acad Dermatol* 1996;35:113–114.

[8]   Butler PD, Longaker MT, Yang GP. Current progress in keloid research and treatment. *J Am Coll Surg*. 2008 Apr;206(4):731-41. Epub 2008 Feb 1.

[9]   van de Kar AL., Kreulen M., van Zuijlen PPM., Oldenburger F. The Results of Surgical Excision and Adjuvant Irradiation for Therapy-Resistant Keloids: A Prospective Clinical Outcome Study. *Plast Reconstr Surg*. 2007 Jun;119(7):2248-54

[10]   Borok TL, Bray M, Sinclair I, et al. Role of ionizing irradiation for 393 keloids. *Int J Radiat Oncol Biol Phys* 1998: 15:836–870.

[11]   Botwood N, Lewanski , Lowdell C The risks of treating keloids with radiotherapy. *Br J Radiol* 1999, 72:1222-24.

[12]   Mettler FA Jr, Hempelmann LH, Dutton AM, Pifer JW, Toyooka ET, Ames WR Breast neoplasms in women treated with x rays for acute postpartum mastitis. A pilot study. *J Natl Cancer Inst*. 1969 Oct;43(4):803-11.

[13]   Metayer C, Lynch CF et All. Second cancers among long-term survivors of Hodgkin's disease diagnosed in childhood and adolescence. *J Clin Oncol*. 2000;18:2435–2443

[14]   Bölke E, Peiper M, Budach W, Matuschek C, Schwarz A, Orth K, Gripp S. Unilateral keloid formation after bilateral breast surgery and unilateral radiation. *Eur J Med Res*. 2007 Jul 26;12(7):320-2

[15] de Lorenzo F, Tielemans H, vd Hulst R, Rhemrev R, Nieman F, Lutgens L, Boeckx W. Is the treatment of Keloids Still a Challenge in 2006? *Annals Plastic Surgery.*2007 Feb;58:186-92.

[16] Devalia H, Mansfield L, Minakaran N, Banerjee D. A case of unilateral keloid after bilateral breast reduction. *Int Semin Surg Oncol.* 2008 Feb 24;5:3.

[17] Hulsbergen Henning JP, Roskam Y, van Gemert MJ. Treatment of keloids and hypertrophic scars with an argon laser. *Lasers Surg Med* 1986;6:72-5.

[18] Norris JE. The effect of carbon dioxide laser surgery on the recurrence of keloids. *Plast Reconstr Surg* 1991;87:44-9.

[19] Paquet P, Hermanns JF, Pierard GE. Effect of the 585 nm flashlamp-pumped pulsed dye laser for the treatment of keloids. *Dermatol Surg* 2001;27:171-4.

[20] Rusciani L, Rossi G, Bono R. Use of cryotherapy in thetreatment of keloids. *J Dermatol Surg Oncol* 1993;19:529-34.

In: Handbook of Skin Care in Cancer Patients   ISBN: 978-1-61668-419-8
Editors: Pierre Vereecken and Ahmad Awada   © 2012 Nova Science Publishers, Inc.

Chapter 13

CYTOTOXIC DRUG EXTRAVASATION IN CANCER PATIENTS: DIAGNOSIS, PREVENTION AND MANAGEMENT

Yassine Lalami

Institut Jules Bordet, Department of Medicine, Medical Oncology Unit,
Oncologic Day Hospital, Rue Héger Bordet, 1. 1000 Bruxelles, Belgium

ABSTRACT

Chemotherapy remains a cornerstone for the treatment of cancer, either for solid and haematological malignancies, in early and advanced stage disease. The very great majority of cytotoxic drugs are administered by intravenous perfusions. Moreover, various toxicities are associated to anticancer chemotherapy, depending on the type of cytotoxic agent considered. Such acute or delayed toxicities are currently well managed, allowing a preservation of patient's quality of life during the scheduled treatment. However, cytotoxic drug extravasation can be considered as an iatrogenic complication well described in the literature, but also probably underestimated and understudied, with a clear lack of general consensus for the medical management, even if practical rules are being developed in clinical institutions.

INTRODUCTION

In oncology practice, extravasation is defined as an inadvertent escape of chemotherapy drug into the extravascular space, secondary to a leakage from a vessel or due to a direct infiltration [1-3]. Even if considered as a rare complication, great variations in the rates of reported incidence, mainly derived from retrospective data, and considered to be between 0.1% and 6.5% for peripheral IV infusions and 0.3-5% in cases of implanted venous access port infusions [4-5]. Such published rates are likely underestimated, as many cases of extravasation remain unreported. However, increasing awareness of complications associated to extravasations and improvement of infusion techniques probably will probably lead to lower incidence. Chemotherapy extravasation is a serious condition warranting special attention from the healthcare professionals, even if the clinical degree of severity of tissue injury is dependent on the chemotherapy agent and the amount injected.

DRUG CLASSIFICATION AND PATHOGENESIS

Cytotoxic drugs can be classified by their potential to cause tissue damage as irritants or vesicants [6-8] (Tables 1-2). An irritant drug will tend to cause pain around the injection site, and will mainly cause inflammatory reaction without tissue necrosis, leading usually to short duration symptoms (burning, tightness, pain and phlebitis) most commonly without long-lasting sequelae. Conversely, a vesicant drugs have the ability to induce blistering and ulceration, causing, if not treated, tissue necrosis with a much more severe and long-lasting local injury, leading to loss of the thickness of skin, and underlying structures. A third group of agents classified as non-vesicants is usually described, including drugs that do not cause ulceration and rarely produce acute reaction or progress to necrosis if extravasated (Table 3). Even among such called non-vesicant drugs, clinicians must consider that any agent extravasatd in high enough concentration may be irritant. Therefore, many antineoplastic agents may overlap such definitions of irritants or vesicants, having the capacity of acting as either, with examples in the literature of absence of tissue necrosis even after vesicant drug extravasation. Indeed, some drugs classified as non-vesicants, irritants, or mild vesicants (e.g., cisplatin, oxaliplatin, paclitaxel, docetaxel, mitoxantrone) have been associated with extravasation injuries [9-15], adding more controversies about the clinical management of such extravasation figures.

Even if not fully understood, data regarding the pathogenesis of such complication is derived from the nature and mechanism of action of the extravasated drug [16-17]. Indeed, vesicant drugs can be sub-classified according the mechanism involved in tissue damage, as DNA binding agents, including anthracyclines (doxorubicin, daunorubicin, epirubicin, mitoxantrone), antitumor antibiotics (mitomycin), and some alkylating agents (mechlorethamine and platinum analogs) and DNA non-binding drugs such vinca alkaloids (vincristine, vinblastine and vinorelbine) and taxanes (paclitaxel and docetaxel). This distinction may explain their highly aggressive effect with variable outcomes after extravasation, which is very important since it affects the management strategy. DNA-binding vesicant drugs are absorbed locally, entering cells and will bind to nucleic acids (DNA), leading to cell death. Thereafter, such DNA-doxorubicin complexes will be taken up by endocytosis in adjacent healthy cells [18]. Such continuous cell damage cycle will induce severe, larger and deeper injuries. Additionally, the significant free radical formation of vesicant agents is suggested as a potential mechanism of the severe necrotic effect. On the other hand, DNA non-binding vesicant drugs will be metabolized in the tissue after extravasation and easily neutralised. So, the damage may remain more localised without devastating effect.

Table 1. Vesicant cytotoxic drugs

DNA-Binding	Non-DNA-Binding
Actinomycin D	Cisplatin (high concentration)
Amsacrine	Dacarbazine
Daunorubicin	Docetaxel
Doxorubicin	Etoposide
Epirubicin	Liposomal doxorubicin
Idarubicin	Mitoxantrone
Mechlorethamine	Oxaliplatin
Mitomycine C	Paclitaxel
	Vinblastine
	Vincristine
	Vindesine
	Vinorelbine

Table 2. Irritant cytotoxic drugs

Bleomycine
Carboplatin
Carmustine
Cyclophosphamide
Cytarabine
Estramustine
Etoposide
Fludarabine
Gemcitabine
Ifosfamide
Irinotecan
Melphalan
Mitoxantrone
Oxaliplatin
Raltitrexed
Streptozocin
Téniposide
Thiotepa
Topotecan

Table 3. Non-vesicant drugs

Cladribine
Cytarabine
Fludarabine
Fluorouracil
Irinotecan
L-Asparaginase
Methotrexate
Raltitrexed

RISK FACTORS

Various risk factors have been reported in the literature, regarding chemotherapy extravasations [4-6]. Beside the treatment-related risk factors (e.g. type of agent, dose, concentration, duration of exposure, administration schedule and frequency), patients receiving cancer therapies may have multiple inherent risk factors that can favour extravasation, including age (very young and aged patients), small and fragile blood vessels (e.g elderly patients), sclerosed veins, obesity, pre-existing conditions (e.g. diabetes, radiation damage, peripheral circulatory conditions, superior vena cava syndrome, lymphedema), cognitive dysfunction with inability to report early symptoms (e.g. sedated, confused patient) and decreased sensation (as a result of peripheral neuropathy). Other risk factors may be associated with cannulation and infusion procedure, equipment, including use of steel butterfly needle rather than plastic cannula, CVC-specific issues, and infusion maintenance. Extravasations from CVC may appear secondary to catheter thrombosis (3-3.5%), catheter fracture, disconnection (0.5%) or dislocation (1.5%-2% of cases) [19-20].

Finally, clinician-related risk factors should also be taken into consideration in this situation. Indeed, nurses must have excellent chemotherapy knowledge and skills, with a perfect application of good clinical practice rules during chemotherapy infusions [8]. Such attitude will allow the performance of comprehensive assessments and identification of early indicators of possible extravasation, and thus appropriate interventions.

CLINICAL MANIFESTATIONS

Extravasation of nonvesicant drugs generally does not cause tissue damage, whereas an irritant drug will cause moderate inflammation at the site of injection, along the vein: aching, swelling, pain or phlebitis. Sclerosis and hyperpigmentation may appear, among burning, local pain, erythema and tenderness. However, these symptoms are self-limiting without long-term sequelae [3-4].

Early symptoms and signs of extravasation from a vesicant drug are often subtle, appearing either early or being delayed for days to weeks [5-6]. Initial symptom is usually a local burning at the infusion site, erythema and swelling. In the following days will appear more diffused erythema, pain, eschar formation, induration and dry desquamation with or without blistering. With more extensive infiltrations, necrosis and ulcerations will appear. Published patients series have estimated that approximately one third of vesicant extravasations will progress to tissue ulceration. Such ulcerations are usually lacking of granulation tissue with little peripheral re-epithelisation. More severe clinical features will involve destruction of underlying tendons, nerves and vessels, leading to various sequelae such as nerve compression, permanent joint stiffness, contractures and peripheral neurologic dysfunction. Central venous catheter extravasation can be complicated by local skin tissue necrosis in the chest wall and the neck, severe pain, effusions, dysrythmias or mediastinitis that can be life threatening [21-22]. Some cases of squamous cell skin carcinoma have been reported as a late complication of chronic extravasation ulcerations [23].

Extravasations must be distinguished from flare reactions, defined as a self-limiting hypersensitivity reaction along peripheral veins, without edema and loss of blood return. It is a rare situation observed in 3% of treatments with anthracyclines or mechlorethamine. Such perturbating reaction must lead to the interruption of the infusion, since it can be confusing for the nurse to differentiate it from an extravasation episode [24].

Recall phenomenon Isa rare phenomenon that has been described with paclitaxel, docetaxel, doxorubicin and epirubicin, consisting in an inflammation reaction occuring after re-exposure to the same extravasated drug administered at a remote IV site. The mechanism of action is currently unknown. The most well-known recall phenomenon is radiation recall causing other types of recall dermatitis rare reactions [25-26].

Beside such esthetical and functional disorders, patients are facing the stress of treatment delays that can impair with the disease clinical outcome. Moreover, extravasation can lead to longer hospital stay, more consultations and increased length of follow up, and higher costs for the society [27]. This can be very difficult to be accepted and managed by the patient and families, especially in an adjuvant setting. In several cases, severe extravasations injury experiences have led patients to change their healthcare provider, due to a loss of confidence.

PREVENTIVE GUIDELINES

The most important approach to extravasation is prevention [28-31]. Several major factors that must be considered to minimize the potential of extravasations are summarized here;

- Use of a large and well selected vein with good blood return before the start of infusion.
- Order of preference for infusion sites: basilic, cephalic and median antebrachial (forearm), dorsum of the hand, wrist, antecubital fossae. In case of breast surgery followed by lymph node resection, there are still controversies about the necessity to avoid IV lines on the ipsilateral side. In daily practice, only the contra-lateral arm continues to be used for chemotherapy perfusions.
- Drugs should never be administered using a butterfly needle; a catheter has always to be inserted into the vein.
- During the infusion, patients should be closely monitored for pain and the site inspected for erythema and swelling.
- Despite their potential complications, use of subcutaneous central venous catheter device should be preferred in case of long-term treatment with vesicant agents. Clinicians and nurses must be aware that such device does not confer an absolute protection against extravasations. Indeed, rate of extravasations from subcutaneous ports have been described to be similar to that reported for peripheral lines (6-7%).
- Clinicians should not permit the use of implanted port in case of absence of blood return, even in cases of easy flush by nurses. In such cases, further investigations are needed. Especially among outpatients, placement in lateral decubitus or in a supine position may allow the observation of blood return. Clinicians should consider the instillation of thrombolytic agent (e.g, tissue plasminogen activator) when partial or total occlusion occurs [32]. A simple chest x-ray can ascertain the right position of CVC devices and exclude any fractured material or dislocation.

- Healthcare professionals must admit and accept the occurrence of an extravasation episode, even in settings of highly experienced oncology nurses treating patients in cancer centres.

- Written guidelines for the management of cytotoxic agent's extravasations should be present in any departments using such drugs. Moreover, clinicians and nurses must have access to an extravasation kit, containing all the material and quick recommendations following the incriminated drug. Finally, any episode of extravasation has to be reported to the institution authorities.

- An adequate and complete patient and family teaching program should be performed, allowing a close collaboration from patients receiving ambulatory continuous IV vesicant chemotherapy, as well as for those who return at home after treatment in clinics with vesicant agents. In case of suspicion of extravasation, an adequate follow up will be crucial to define exactly the diagnosis and to propose adapted therapeutic strategies.

CLINICAL DIAGNOSIS OF EXTRAVASATION

It is crucial that an extravasation is recognised and diagnosed early. Healthcare profesionnals must be aware of any early reported symptoms and clinical signs, and must be ready to act promptly [3-4, 7-8]. Moreover, it will also be very important to rule out other possible clinical conditions, such as flare reactions. Patient's reporting symptoms are crucial, and the healthcare team must encourage patients to report any symptom during the infusion (such as pain, swelling redness, burning, and discomfort). Even if such complaints may lack for specificity of extravasation, they should be treated with concern and warrant further examination (testing the patency of infusion with blood return control). Once again, clinicians must keep in mind that such symptoms and signs may appear later in the extravasation process. A careful verification of the infusion line (peripheral or central) is probably the more useful technique to confirm any suspected extravasation. Alarming clinical signs that must be considered are the lack or loss of blood return from the cannula, any change in infusion flow and increased resistance during the administration of IV drugs. In such situation, the cannula should be removed, and replaced in other vein (ideally above the previous injection site).

As reported earlier, distinction between extravasation and other local reactions is crucial for final diagnosis and subsequent clinical management. Beside flare reactions, already described, other potential conditions include vessel infiltration, phlebitis, vessel irritation and hypersensitivity.

TREATMENT OF EXTRAVASATIONS

Because of a lack of controlled studies in humans, most of available informations for such management are derived from animal models, case reports and small limited uncontrolled trials [33-35]. It is important to note that delays in recognition and treatment can increase the risk of tissue necrosis in case of vesicants extravasations Moreover, local procedures and protocols are crucial for an optimal management [8]. Even if there is a clear lack of international consensus, several examples of existing policies and protocols are available online. Since every vesicant extravasation is unique; the type of therapeutic approach will be influenced by the type of extravasated vesicant (DNA versus non-DNA binding), drug concentration, amount in the tissue and finally, the location of the injury.

PHARMACOLOGIC MANAGEMENT

First, and no matter what the nature of the drug, the first course of action is to stop and disconnect the infusion, to aspirate as much as possible from the cannula, to mark the affected area and finally and finally, remove the cannula. It is advised to elevate the affected limb and to administer analgesia if required. In an ideal situation, a digital picture of the affected area should be performed at the moment of diagnosis and, in the following days, to illustrate the clinical evolution. General measures can be taken to limit inflammation, discomfort and pain (antihistamines and analgesics). The real place of topical corticosteroids in that setting remains controversial, since it was shown that only few inflammatory cells are found in damaged tissues. Moreover, topical corticoid application appears to be ineffective, and may lead to increased skin ulceration. Conversely, oral dexamethasone treatment allowed a reduction of inflammatory reaction associated with oxaliplatin extravasation [11-13].

Further clinical management will depend on the nature of extravasated drug. Various clinical small sample sized studies have reported the potential benefit of saline lavage and suction techniques (wash-out), avoiding surgical debridment in various cases of vesicant extravasations, and appearing to be superior to the watch and await approach [36-37]. The success of this technique is attributed to the dilution and removal of extravasated vesicant agents from the injured area.

HEAT OR COLD APPLICATION?

Local applications of cold or heat have been used empirically for years [5-6]. Hot packs are believed to cause vasodilatation, increasing of blood flow, leading to the dilution of extravasated drug and enhancement of drug removal. Cold packs will induce vasoconstriction with localization of the drugs and increasing the degradation of toxic metabolites and reducing the extent of local injury. Moreover, cooling may reduce local inflammation and pain. Intermittent 15 minutes applications every 4 hours during 24-48 hours are usually recommended.

In practice, cold application is recommended for extravasation of all vesicant or irritant drugs except the vinca alkaloids (vincristine, vinblastine, vinorelbine) and epipodophyllotoxins such as etoposide.

In case of taxanes extravasations, the role of heat versus cold is less clear [9-10, 38]. Most guidelines suggest the application of ice for paclitaxel extravasations, long-term effects in such case being minimal with mild fibrosis in the incriminated. Conversely, skin toxicity with desquamation is more frequent with docetaxel extravasation. The relative benefit of topical cooling for docetaxel extravasations is less clear than for paclitaxel; some authors suggesting the use of heat in such cases.

ANTIDOTES

Historically, various medications and substances have been injected or topically applied to vesicant extravasation injuries during the last three decades, but only limited breakthroughs have been achieved [39]. Many of these drugs, such as glucocorticoids, hydrocortisone, antihistamines, sodium bicarbonate and lidocain have been found to be ineffective in such therapeutic setting. Other agents (e.g. alpha tocopherol) have been somewhat effective, but only in limited case report series. The growth factor, GM-CSF, was shown to be effective in accelerating wound healing without the need for skin grafts [40-41]. Moreover, such findings appeared to be difficult to apply in clinical practice since many of these drugs were administered with concurrent treatments such as systemic or topical antibiotics.

Antidotes are agents used with the aim to neutralise the cytotoxic effect of the infiltrated agent, usually vesicants. Most pertinent clinical data are derived from four main antidotes currently available for the treatment of extravasations: dexrazoxane (Savene), dimethylsulfoxide (DMSO), sodium thiosulfate and hyaluronidase (Table 4).

Table 4. Antidotes for extravasations treatments

Cytotoxic agent	Antidotes	Procedures
Anthracyclines	DMSO 50%	Topical application, every 6-8h for 7-14 days.
	Topical cooloing	Immediate 30-60 min, then every 15 min for 1 day .
	Dexrazoxane	IV within 6 hours of extravasation in the opposite site: $1000mg/m^2$ on day1 and 2; $500 mg/m^2$ on day 3.
Liposomal anthracyclines	Topical cooling	
Vinca alkaloids	Warm compress	Immediate, then on/off for 1day.
Epipodophyllotoxins	Hyaluronidase	150U/ml; SC Injection 1-6ml (150- 900U) into the extravasation site through the existing line.
Mitomycin C	DMSO 50%	Same as for anthracyclines
Taxanes	Topical cooling Hyaluronidase	Same as vinca alkaloids
Mechlorethamine Concentrated cisplatin	Sodium thiosulfate 1/6 mol/L (isotonic)	Immediate SC injection at extravasation site : 4 ml of 10% sodium thiosulfate and 6 ml sterile water for injection.
Other agents		Topical cooling

DMSO: dimethylsulfoxide; IV: intranenous; SC: subcutaneous.

Sodium thiosulfate prevents alkylation and subsequent subcutaneous tissue destruction by providing a substrate for alkylation. Local injection is recommended for the treatment of mechlorethamine (nitrogen mustard) extravasations, as well as for large volume extravasation of dacarbazine or cisplatin. Sodium thiosulfate appears to neutralise mechlorethamine to form non-toxic thioesters that will be excreted in urine [42]. Once again, such recommendations are largely based on in vitro data. Clinical benefit among patients with mechlorethamine extravasation is poorly documented in a single case report [43]. Mean healing time also appeared to be improved with sodium thiosulfate (2% solution injected subcutaneously) in patients with extravasations from doxorubicin, epirubicin, vinblastine or mitomycin C, when compared to standard management with hydrocortisone and dexamethasone [31].

DMSO is known to enhance the skin permeability, which may facilitate systemic absorption of extrvasated agents. Topical application of DMSO prevents ulceration by its free radical scavenging property, and has been recommended by some groups for anthracyclines and mitomycin extravasation [44]. Such recommendations were derived from at least two observational studies. In the largest study, a dual application of local cooling therapy (60 minutes every 8 hours for three days) and topical DMSO (application of 99% solution every 8 hours for seven days) allowed a complete clinical recovery within one week in 71% of patients (103/144 pts), while 22 others needed more than a week to recover total success rate of 87%) [45]. Main criticism for such data interpretation came from the fact that those patients received upfront a combined therapy and, furthermore, only 62 extravasations were due to known vesicant drugs, while the remainder involved irritant drugs. A further limited, but more homogeneous phase II study, investigated the potential benefit of DMSO without cooling application in 20 pts with anthracycline extravasations. None of these patients developed ulceration or required surgical management. DMSO side effects reported are erythema, itching, mild burning sensation and a characteristic breath odor [46]. Despite these findings, many questions remain unsolved about the real mechanism of action and the optimal dose and duration of treatment. Moreover, several international guidelines, including the Oncology Nursing Society, do not include DMSO in their recommendations.

Hyaluronidase is a proteolytic enzyme that is thought to break down hyaluronic acid in connective tissue stroma, allowing a dispersion of the extravasated drug with reduction of local concentration and increase of absorption [47]. It is postulated that this creates a wider surface for dilution and aspiration of the drug. Its clinical impact lie on the results of two small clinical reports, concluding that local infiltration of hyaluronidase may be recommended in case of extravasations of vinca alkaloids, paclitaxel, epipodophyllotoxins and ifosfamide [48-49]. The recommended dose is 1 ml (150 units) infiltrated subcutaneously.

Finally, dexrazoxane is actually the only registered antidote for anthracyclines extravasations, acting as a catalytic inhibitor of DNA topoisomerase II (which is the target of anthracyclines), and so, the blocked enzyme is no more affected by antharcyclines and further cell damage is avoided. Its activity in protecting tissue may be explained by the capacity to scavenge free radicals and also, the effect on catalytic cycle of topopisomerase II. Benefit for dexrazoxane after extravasation was initially suggested in animal studies and isolated case reports [50-51]. Dexrazoxane was studied and validated in prevention of anthracyclines induced cardiomyopathy in metastatic breast cancer patient. Final and robust clinical data in the field of extravasation came from two recent prospective nonrandomized multicenter studies pooled for analysis, involving 80 pts with suspected antharcycline extravasations [52].

Such complication has been confirmed by fluorescence microscopy of a biopsy specimen in 54 evaluable cases. Dexrazoxane (Totect[R], Savene[R]) was administered intravenously in a large vein in an area away from the extravasation site (e.g. the opposite arm) as a 1-2 hours infusion, within six hours of the event, and 24 and 48 hours after extravasation. The first and second doses were 1000 mg/m^2 (day s 1 and 2) and the third was 500 mg/m^2 (day 3). Only one patient (2%) required surgical debridment for non-resolving tissue injury. Mild pain (19%) and sensory disturbances (17%) were the most frequent sequelae. Chemotherapy could be continued without interruption in 71% of the cases. Since dexrazoxane is a cytotoxic drug, side effects that were seen are quite comparable to those encountered after anthracyclines infusions, including nausea/ vomiting (19%), diarrhea (4%), stomatitis (4%), bone marrow suppression (neutropenia), transient elevatation of liver enzymes levels (25%) and infusion site reaction (28%). Based upon these results, dexrazoxane was registred and approved in September 2007 by the EMEA and FDA for the treatment of anthracycline extravasation injury. There is currently no other therapeutic equivalent to Totect. It is interesting to observe that none of the patients evaluated in these clinical trials had an extravasation from an implanted port venous catheter [53]. Therefore, further investigation about the efficacy of dexrazoxane in that population would be of great interest.

SURGICAL MANAGEMENT

The optimal timing for surgical salvage remains controversial and surgery should not be considered as the initial treatment of choice [54-57]. Indeed, ulcerative lesions caused by vesicant drugs such anthracyclines are common in about one third of all cases. However, a progression of ulceration and continuing pain will promote a surgical intervention to excise the damaged tissue. Moreover, surgical approach may restore function and reduce the pain in the affected area. Because of their ability to bind to fat tissue, early debridement has been recommended by some authors for anthracycline extravasations. This was based on a small serie of three cases in which delayed surgical management led to impaired functional outcome. Such debridement is usually completed by wound closure with skin graft.

Fluorescein guidance is considered as an interesting diagnostic tool for the observation of the extension from extravasations injuries and may be helpful for the surgical indication [58-60]. It has been shown that local injection of IV fluorescein into doxorubicin extravasation allowed the identification of non-necrotic tissue, since anthracyclines exhibit fluorescence under UV light. Thereafter, surgical removal of residual necrotic tissue without fluorescence was performed. Clinical cases of fluorescence negative specimens did not develop tissue necrosis. In Europe, surgical resection is immediate if biopsies from the area of extravasation are fluorescent, and such area can be observed in case of negative biopsies. In a Danish report, among 22 patients suspected pf having an anthracycline extravasation, nine patients whose biopsies were negative for fluorescence were observed without intervention and none showed sequelae [58]. However, among the 13 fluorescence-positive pts who underwent surgery, eight of them presented sequelae such as atrophy, skin ulceration and dysmobility. Moreover, surgery may cause subsequent delays in chemotherapy schedule until adequate and complete healing of the wound.

Controversial data were derived from a recent observational study in which all of the 18 pts who were referred later to surgeons (mean of 22 days after extravasation) required debridement. The authors concluded that early surgery may reduce the need for complex surgical procedures [61]. Finally, magnetic resonance imaging (MRI) can be used to estimate the deep soft tissue damage, leading to appropriate surgical treatment [62].

CONCLUSION

Despite all preventive efforts, cytotoxic drug extravasations still occur in clinical practice. Close multidisciplinary collaboration is precious for an optimal management, since it is performed in accordance with the latest scientific understanding and medical consensus following protocols and local policies. Clinicians who administer vesicant agents must demonstrate appropriate skills and knowledge regarding the recognition and management of extravasation. Despite recent limited phase II studies, management of extravasations still remains based on anecdotal efficacy of interventions from single clinical cases. In the future, there will be a strong need for international collaboration, allowing establishment of reinforced guidelines, after systematic data collection and case reporting, allowing a further development of evidence-based patient care.

As mentioned earlier and after three decades of research and clinical studies, clinicians have now access to dexrazoxane, considered as the first and unique IV antidote to antharcyclines extravasations, showing the highest reported efficacy rate (98%) in clinical trials. Such agent must be used safely in a precise timing and schedule of administration. Unfortunately, it is not indicated and not effective for the treatment of other types of vesicant extravasatiuons such vinca alkaloids, alkylating agents and taxanes. Moreover and despite such a precious help, clinicians and nurses must not negate the need for more extravasation prevention efforts.

In clinical practice, the widespread use of central venous catheter ports in cancer patients must not be considered as an absolute protection against the potential risk of extravasation. As reported earlier, CVC extravasation can lead to devastating and life-threatening injuries. This population should be considered for further clinical studies, allowing a better comprehension and optimal management schedule. The role of dexrazoxane in such indication still needs to be defined.

Finally, a better comprehension of carcinogenesis allowed the emergence of various molecular targeted therapies. Since the majority of these drugs are being administered intravenously, alone or in combination with cytotoxic chemotherapy, careful observation and poroposal of management are warranted in clinical practice. Only few data are available about the vesicant potential of such new anticancer drugs.

REFERENCES

[1]   Bach F, Holst-Christensen J, Boesby S. Cytostatic extravasation. *Cancer* 1991; 68:538-539.

[2]   How C, Brown J. Extravasation of cytotoxic chemotherapy from peripheral veins. *Eur J Oncol Nurs* 1998; 2(1): 51-58.

[3]   Susser WS, Whitacker-Worth DL, Grant-Kels JM. Mucocutaneous reactions to chemotherapy. *Acad Dermatol* 1999; 40:367-398.

[4]   Schrijvers DL. Extravasation: a dreaded complication of chemotherapy. *Ann Oncol* 2003; 14 (S3): 26-30.

[5]   McCaffey Boyle D Engelking C. Vesicant extravasation: myths and realities. *Oncol Nurs Forum* 1995; 22(1):57-67.

[6]   Ener RA, Meglathery SB, Styler M. Extravasation of systemic hemato-oncological therapies. *Ann Oncol* 2004; 15:858-862.

[7]   Sanborn RE, Sauer DA. Cutaneous reactions to chemotherapy: commonly seen, less described, little understood. *Dermatol Clin* 2008; 26:103-119.

[8]   Polovich M, White J, Kelleher L. (Eds) *Chemotherapy and biotherapy guidelines and recommendations for practice.* 2005 (2nd.Ed); Pittsburgh, PA: Oncology Nursing Society.

[9]   Stanford BL, Hardwicke F. A review of clinical experience with paclitaxel extravasations. *Support Care Cancer* 2003; 11:270-277.

[10]   Berghammer P, Pohln R, Baur M et al. Docetaxel extravasation. *Support Care Cancer* 2001;9:131-134.

[11]   Kretzschmar A, Pink D, Thuss-Patience P et al. Extravasations of oxaliplatin. *J Clin Oncol* 2003; 21:4068-4069.

[12]   Kennedy JG, Donahue JP, Hoang P et al. Vesicant characteristics of oxaliplatin following antecubital extravasation. *Clin Oncol* 2003; 15:237-239.

[13]   Foo KF, Michael M, Toner G et al. A case report of oxaliplatin extravasation (Letter). *Ann Oncol* 2003; 14:961-962.

[14]   Luke E. Mitoxantrone-induced extravasation. *Oncol Nurs Forum* 2005; 32:27-29.

[15]   Patel JS. Distant and delayed mitomycin C extravasation. *Pharmacother* 1999; 19(8): 1002-1005.

[16]   Sauerland C, Engelking C, Wickham R et al. Vesicant extravasations part I: mechanisms, pathogenesis, and nursing care to reduce risk. *Oncol Nurs Forum* 2006; 33(6): 1134-1141.

[17]   Rudolph R, Larson DL. Etiology and treatment of chemotherapeutic agent extravasation injuries: a review. *J Clin Oncol* 1987; 5(7): 1116-1126.

[18]   Reeves D. Management of anthracycline extravasation injuries. *Ann Pharmacother* 2007; 41(7): 1238-1242.

[19]   Lemmers NW, Gels ME, Sleijfer DT et al. Complications of venous access ports in 132 patients with disseminated testicular cancer treated with polychemotherapy. *J Clin Oncol* 1996; 14:2916-2922.

[20]   Goossens S, Jerome M, Stas M. Occlusion in totally implantable vascular access devices: what its incidence and what actions do nurses take to restore patency? 2005. Available   at   http://www.uzleuven.be/ UZRoot/files/webeditor/poster_katherzorg.pdf. Accessed September 26, 2007.

[21]   Schulmeister L, Camp-Sorrell D. Chemotherapy extravasation from implanted ports. *Oncol Nurs Forum* 2000; 27(3): 539-540.

[22]   Bozkurt AK, Uzel B, Akman C et al. Intrathoracic extravasation of antineoplastic agents: case reports and systematic review. *Am J Clin Oncol* 2003; 26:121-123.

[23]   Lauvin R, Miglianico L, Hellegouarc'h R. Skin cancer occurring 10years after the extravasation of doxorubicin (Letter). *N Engl J Med* 1995; 332:754.

[24]   Curran CF, Luce JK. Doxorubicin-associated flare reactions. *Oncol Nurs Forum* 119; 17:387-389.

[25] Shapiro J, Richardson GE. Paclitaxel-induced "recall" soft tissue injury occurring at the site of previous extravasation with subsequent intravenous treatment in a different limb. *J Clin Oncol* 1994; 12:2237-2238.

[26] Diaz-Levy B, Sanchez Perez J, Fraga J et al. Recall Phenomenon in site of previous drug extravasation. *J Am Acad Dermatol* 2008; abstract P439.

[27] Weiner MG, Ross SJ, Mathew JL et al. Estimating the costs of chemotherapy-associated adverse event clusters. *Health Serv Outcomes res Method 2007,* In print.

[28] Hadaway LC. Preventing and managing peripheral extravasation. *Nursing* 2004; 34(5): 66-67.

[29] Goolsby TV and Lombardo FA. Extravasation of chemotherapeutic agents: prevention and treatment. *Semin Oncol* 2006; 33(1): 139-143.

[30] Bertelli G. Prevention and management of extravasation of cytotoxic drugs. *Drug Saf* 1995; 12(4): 245-255.

[31] Tsavaris NB, Komitsopoulou P, Karagiaouris P et al. Prevention of tissue necrosis due to accidental extravasation of cytotoxic drugs by a conservative approach. *Cancer Chemother Pharmacol* 1992; 30:330-333.

[32] Ponec D, Irwin D, Haire WD et al. Recombinant tissue plasminogen activator (ateplase) for restoration of flow in occluded central venous access devices: a double-blind placebo-controlled trial – the Cardiovascular Thrombolytic to Open Occluded lines (COOL) efficacy trial. *J Vasc Interv Radiol* 2001; 12:951-955.

[33] Schulmeister L. Managing vesicant extravasations. *Oncologist* 2008; 13: 284-288.

[34] Schulmeister L. Extravasation management. *Semin Oncol Nurs 2007*; 23 (3):184-190.

[35] Wickham R, Engelking C, Sauerland C et al. Vesicant extravasation part II: evidence-based management and continuing controversies. *Oncol Nurs Forum* 2006; 33(6): 1143-1150.

[36] Vandeweyer E, Deraemaecker R. Early surgical suction and washout for treatment of cytotoixic drug extravasations. *Acta Chir Belg* 1994; 100:37-38.

[37] Giunta R. Early subcutaneous wash-out in acute extravasations *Ann Oncol* 2004; 15:1146.

[38] Ascherman JA, Knowles SL, Attkiss K. Docetaxel (taxotere) extravasation: a report of five cases with treatment recommendations. *Ann Plast Surg* 2000; 45:438-441.

[39] Door RT. Antidotes to vesicant extravasations. *Blood Rev* 1990; 4:41-60.

[40] Saghir NE, Otrock Z, Muffarij A et al. Dexrazoxane for anthracycline extravasation and GM-CSF for skin ulceration and wound healing. *Lancet Oncol* 2004; 5:320-321.

[41] Ulutin HC, Guden M, Dede M et al. Comparison of granulocyte-colony stimulating factor and granulocyte macrophage-colony stimulating factor in the treatment of chemotherapy extravasation ulcers. *Eur J Gynaecol Oncol* 2000; 21:613-615.

[42] Dorr RT, Soble M,Alberts DS. Efficacy of sodium thiosulfate as a local antidote to mechlorethamine skin toxicity in the mouse. *Cancer Chemother Pharmacol* 1988; 22:299-302.

[43] Owen OE, Dellatorre DL, Van Scott EJ et al. Accidental intramuscular injection of mechlorethamine *Cancer* 1980; 45:2225-2226.

[44] Guidelines on management of chemotherapy extravasation. *American Society of Health-System Pharmacists*.www.ashp.org

[45] Bertelli G, Gozza A, Forno GB et al. Topical dimethylsulfoxide for the prevention of soft tissue injury after extravasation of vesicant cytotoxic drugs: a prospective clinical study. *J Clin Oncol* 1995; 13:2851-2855.

[46] Olver IN, Aisner J, Hament A et al. A prospective study of topical dimethyl sulfoxide for treating anthracycline extravasation. *J Clin Oncol* 1988; 6:1732-....

[47] Dorr RT, Alberts DS. Vinca alkaloid skin toxicity: antidote and drug disposition studies in the mouse. *J Natl Cancer Inst* 1985; 47:113-120.

[48] Bertelli G, dini D, Forno GB et al. Hyaluronidase as an antidote to extravasation of vinca alkaloids: clinical results. *J Cancer Res Clin Oncol* 1994; 120:505-506.

[49] Cicchetti S, Jemec B, Gault DT. Two case reports of vinorelbine extravasation: management and review of the literature. *Tumori* 2000; 86:289-292.

[50] Langer SW, Sehested M, Buhl Jensen P. Dexrazoxane is a potent and specific inhibitor of anthracycline induced subcutaneous lesions in mice. *Ann Oncol* 2001; 12:405-410.

[51] Langer SW, Sehested M, Buhl Jensen P. Treatment of anthracycline extravasation with dexrazoxane. *Clin Cancer Res* 2000; 6:3680-3686.

[52] Mouridsen HT, Langer SW, Buter J et al. Treatment of anthracycline extravasation with Savene (dexrazoxane): results from two prospective clinical multicentre studies. *Ann Oncol* 2007; 18:546-550.

[53] Kane RC, McGuinn Jr WD, Dagher R et al. Dexrazoxane (Totect TM): FDA review and approval for the treatment of accidental extravasation following intravenous anthracycline chemotherapy. *Oncologist* 2008; 13:445-450.

[54] Heckler FR. Current thoughts on extravasation injuries. *Clin Plast Surg* 1989; 16:557-563.

[55] Scuderi N, Onesti MG. Antitumor agents: extravasation, management, and surgical treatment. *Ann Plast Surg* 1994; 32:39-44.

[56] D'Andrea F, Onesti MG, Nicoletti GF et al. Surgical treatment of ulcers caused by extravasation of cytotoxic drugs. *Scand J Plast Reconstr Surg Hand Surg.* 2004; 38(5): 288-292.

[57] Heitmann C, Durmus C, Ingianni G. Surgical management after doxorubicin and epirubicin extravasation. *J Hand Surg* 1998; 22:666-668.

[58] Andersson AP, Dahlstrom KK. Clinical results after doxorubicin extravasation treated with excision guided by fluorescence microscopy. *Eur J Cancer* 1993;29:1712-1714.

[59] Dahlstrom KK, Chenoufi HL, Daugaard S. Fluorescence microscopic demonstration and demarcation of doxorubicin extravasation. Experimental and clinical studies. *Cancer* 1990; 65:1722-1726.

[60] Cohen FJ, Manganaro J, Bezozo RC. Identification of involved tissue during surgical treatment of doxorubicin-induced extravasation necrosis. *J Hand Surg* 1983; 8:43-45.

[61] Cedici C, Hierner R, Berger A. Plastic surgical management in tissue extravasation of cytotoxic agents in the upper extremity. *Eur J Med Res* 2001; 6:309-314.

[62] Yama N, Tsuchida Y, Nuka s et al. Usefulness of magnetic resonance imaging for surgical Management of extravasation of an antitumor agent: a case report. *Jpn J Clin Oncol* 2001; 31 (3): 122-124.

In: Handbook of Skin Care in Cancer Patients   ISBN: 978-1-61668-419-8
Editors: Pierre Vereecken and Ahmad Awada   © 2012 Nova Science Publishers, Inc.

Chapter 14

SKIN MANIFESTATIONS OF PARANEOPLASTIC SYNDROMES

Jean Klastersky[1], Maria-Letizia Cappelletti[2], Florence Neczyporenko[2] and Marie-Therese Genot[1]

[1]Institut Jules Bordet, Centre des Tumeurs de l'Université Libre de Bruxelles, Brussels, Belgium
[2]Department of Dermatology, St Pierre-Brugmann-HUDERF, Université Libre de Bruxelles, Belgium

ABSTRACT

Acrokeratosis paraneoplastica, hypertrichosis lanuginosa, erythema gyratum repens, hypertrophic osteoarhtropathy, dermatomyositis and Sweet's syndrome are often – although not always- associated with a malignant tumor. Recognition of any of these potential paraneoplastic skin disorders should lead to a strong suspicion for an occult malignancy and trigger appropriate work-up. In case of negative investigation, a high suspicion level for an occult malignancy must be maintained for years.

Paraneoplastic skin manifestations with well known pathophysiological mechanisms related to a tumor, such as cutaneous amyloidosis, melanic pigmentation, vasculitis, carcinoid flushing, hirsutism, gynecomastia and others, can be responsible for signs and symptoms requiring specific therapies. These manifestations ususally follow a course that is clearly related to that of the tumor and can thus serve as surrogates for its evolution.

INTRODUCTION

Dermatologic diseases are defined as paraneoplastic when they occur in increased frequency in patients with cancer and are not related to a direct effect of tumor, infection or toxicity of therapy. In these situations, the pathophysiological mechanisms underlying the effect of the tumor on the skin manifestations remain unknown in most cases [1,2].

Whether skin manifestations, due to a metabolic abnormality induced by the tumor, should be called paraneoplastic is debatable from the semantic point of view. In these cases, the pathophysiology linking the tumor to the skin manifestations is usually well established, and thus the dermatological syndrome can be seen as an uncommon expression of a tumor. Because these clinical presentations are more frequent than true paraneoplastic syndromes, and also because they have often a specific diagnostic significance, we will discuss these skin manifestations of cancer as well

Table 1. Dermatologic paraneoplastic manifestations of some hereditary disorders

Leukemia, lymphomas	• Recurrent infections, eczema (Wiskott-Aldrich, Bruton) • Recurrent pyoderma (Chediak-Higashi) • Hyperpigmentation (Fanconi) • Teleangectasis (Ataxia-Teleangectasia, Bloom)
Neurological malignancies	• Scleroderma, Progeria (Werner) • Hemangioma (Sturge-Weber) • Pigmented macules,Fibromas (Von Recklinghausen, Bourneville) • Basal cell carcinomas (Gorlin)
Gastro-intestinal cancers Breast - thyroid cancers	• Sebaceous cysts, Lipomas, Fibromas (Gardner) • Mucocutaneous pigmentation (Peutz-Jeghers) • Keratosis (palmo-plantar) (Tylosis) • Keratosis (palmo-plantar), Facial nodules (trichilemmomas) (Cowden)

On the other hand, we will not include in the present review skin neoplasias such as Paget's disease or the Muir Torr syndrome (sebaceous gland neoplasm that may precede, follow or co-exist with visceral cancers) or metastases. The main hereditary disorders associated with cutaneous manifestations of malignancy are summarized in Table 1 and will not be discussed further.

PARANEOPLASTIC SKIN SYNDROMES FROM UNKNOWN CAUSE

The most important such syndromes are presented in Table 2.

For these true paraneoplastic syndromes, it should be stressed, in addition, that benign form exists, that the skin manifestations may precede the cancer signs and/or symtoms and that the dermatological syndrome may or may not regress with cancer response to therapy. There is, overall, little evidence of a specific association for most of these paraneoplastic syndromes with one definite neoplasia.

Acanthosis nigricans (Figure 1) is a dark brown to black velvety hyperpigmentation, appearing mainly on the neck (back and side) and axilla and sometimes on groins, anogenitalia, arm folds, submammary and knukkels [3]. Skin shows epidermal thicking with enhanced skin folds (hyperkeratotic ridges) but blurred limits. It is often associated with pruritus. Tripe palms with major thickning and especially pachydermatoglyphy can be associated to acanthosis nigricans which raises the possibility that they may be part of the same syndrom. [4]. Cause is unknown, although it is mainly associated (preceding by months or years or with a parallel course) with adenocarcinomas (stomach, colon, biliary tract, ovary, lung) which might give us some clues about its pathogenesis.

Acanthosis nigricans has also been described in patients with non neoplastic disease, namely in patients with high level of insulin resistance (Kahn's syndrome) or with severe lipodystrophy (Laurence's syndrome).

No specific effective therapies are available for acanthosis or tripe palms but it may resolve when underlying disease is under control.

Table 2. Paraneoplastic skin syndromes which cause is unknown

Skin disease	Associated malignancy (Not exhaustive neither exclusive)
Acanthosis nigricans	Adenocarcinomas (gastric, ovarian)
Leser-Trelat sign	Lymphomas; gastric and mammary cancer
Bazex's syndrome	Squamous cell (oesophagus, head and neck, lung)
Sweet's syndrome	Hematological malignancies
Pyoderma gangrenosum	Lymphomas; skin cancers
Erythema gyratum repens	Lung, breast, digestive cancers
Ichtyosis	Lymphomas, multiple myeloma
Dermatomyositis	Many different tumors
Hypertrichosis lanuginosa	Colon, gallbladder, lung, uterus, bladder cancers
Pruritus	Lymphomas, hematologic malignancies, lung cancer
Exfoliative dermatitis	Cutaneous T cell lymphomas
Pachydermoperiostosis	Lung cancer
Hyperkeratotic papulonodules	Cutaneous T cell lymphomas

The Leser-Trelat sign or syndrome (Figure 2) consists of the sudden appearance and/or rapid increase in the number and size of seborrheic keratoses [5]. As seborrheic keratoses are common, especially in older patients, the specificity of the paraneoplastic nature of this sign is not always easy to establish.

There is no clear specificity with respect to tumor types associated with the Leser-Trelat sign, as it has been observed with a variety of neoplastic diseases: lymphomas, gastric (perhaps the most frequently reported), breast, colon, kidney cancers, and others, including squamous cell carcinomas.

It is not infrequent that the eruptive onset of multiple seborrheic keratoses precedes by several months the diagnosis of a neoplastic disease. The pathophysiology of the Leser-Trelat syndrome is unknown, so far.

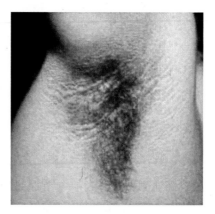

Figure 1. Acanthosis nigricans: black dermal pigmentation.

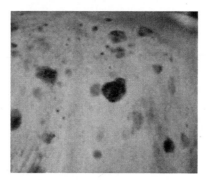

Figure 2. Leser Trelat sign: seborrheic keratosis.

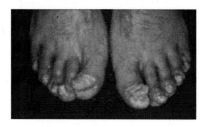

Figure 3. Acrokeratosis paraneoplastica (Bazex's syndrome).

Lesions are benign and do not require specific therapy, however they can be removed for esthetic purpose.

Bazex's syndrome or acrokeratosis paraneoplastica: (Figure 3) consists of a symmetric psoriasiform scaling hyperkeratosis of extremities: mainly hands and feet (typically associated with early ungueal dystrophy that can be severe), but also the nose and outer ears. Desquamation thickness is often impressive and fissures are frequently seen [6]. Skin manifestations can also extend proximally (arms, legs, trunc) or to other extremities and prominent body parts (scalp, elbow, knee, genitalia). Male are much more often affected than female.

Basex's syndrome is mainly associated with squamous cell carcinomas of the esophagus, head and neck and lung. In most cases, by the time of Bazex's syndrome diagnosis, the tumor is already large, with lymph nodes metastases. The syndrome can also precede malignancy diagnosis. Most of the time it improves with successful underlying cancer therapy. In some cases additional local steroids may be of help. Although, pathogenesis is not firmly established, it has been suspected that a cross-reaction between the basement membrane and tumor antigens might play a role, as well as the secretion of various growth factors by the tumor.

Sweet's syndrome (Figure 4) is an acute nodular dermatitis, consisting of painful sharply bordered inflammatory lesions, mainly asymmetrically located on the face, neck and arms. Fever and malaise are usually present and, in some cases, buccal ulcerations and/or lesions resembling erythema nodosum can be present [7, 8].

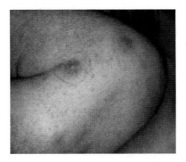

Figure 4. Sweet's syndrome: neutrophilic skin infiltration.

Sweet's syndrome lesions, are histologically characterized by neutrophilic infiltrates and which etiology is thought to be hypersensitivity, as response to corticoids is often rapid.

Sweet's syndrome is associated with malignancy in 20% of the cases; it may precede the neoplasia, sometimes by many years or around the same time. The most common malignancy associated with Sweet's syndrome is acute myelogenous leukemia. Associations with myeloproliferative and lymphoproliferative diseases, myelodysplasic syndromes and solid tumors have also been reported.

Among the non neoplastic diseases associated with Sweet's syndrome, inflammatory diseases such as Crohn's disease have been reported as well as infections, like toxoplasmosis or those caused by Yersinia sp.. In case of associated infection, management includes appropriate antibiotherapy. It can also occur during the course of normal pregnancy. Nonetheless, in most cases (70%) syndrome is idiopathic, with no identified cause.

Pyoderma gangrenosum (Figure 5) appears suddenly, as a papule or a nodule quickly evolving to a very painful purulent necrotic ulcer with undermined and violaceous borders. Fever and malaise are usually present. Histologic examination has some similarities with Sweet's syndrome and shows a neutrophilic infiltration accounting for the purulent exudate and a vasculitic process, leading to necrosis. [9].

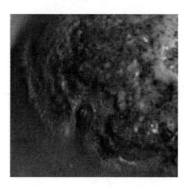

Figure 5. Pyoderma gangrenosum: hemorrhagic necrosis.

It is usually associated with basal and squamous skin cancer as well as with cutaneous lymphomas, other lymphomas amd myeloid disorders. However, pyoderma gangrenosum is chiefly seen in patients with inflammatory bowel disease or rheumatoid arthritis; in these situations, adalimumab (an anti-TNF antibody) has some clinical efficacy.

High doses of glucocorticoids are usually required as well as local care and painkillers.

Erythema gyratum repens or Gammet's syndrome (Figure 6) consists of rapidly progressing concentric rings of scally erythema, sometimes with a vesicular aspect, usually located on trunk and proximal extremities. These lesions are large, flat or slightly raised and extend outwards in a serpiginous pattern (hence the name). Patient often presents with pruritus and marked eosinophilia [10]. There is a strong association with internal malignancies.

Skin lesions precede the neoplasia diagnosis most of the time (80%) and are often associated with lung, breast, uterus and digestive tract malignancies.

Lesions typically regress with therapy of the underlying neoplasia. Local steroids may help in some resistant cases.

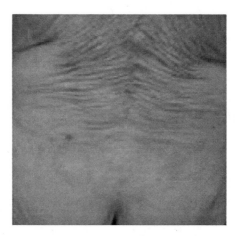

Figure 6. Erythema gyratum repens (Gammet's syndrome): concentric erythema.

Aquired Ichtyosis (Figure 7) typically has a sudden onset and involves the whole body skin which looks dry, with fissures and light rhomboid desquamation. hyperkeratosis is frequently observed [11].

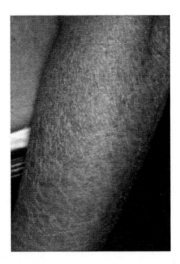

Figure 7. Ichtyosis: hyperkeratosis and desquamation.

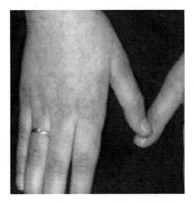

Figure 8. Dermatomyositis: skin appearance.

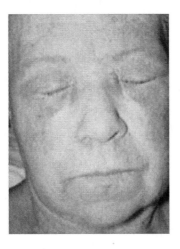

Figure 9. Dermatomyositis: periorbital heliotropic rash.

Ichtyosis is mainly seen in patients with lymphomas (Hodgkin's and non Hodgkin's types); it has also been reported in multiple myeloma, Kaposi's sarcoma and various solid tumors. It is often diagnose at the same time or after the discovery of the tumor and runs a parallel course to that of the neoplasia.

Acquired ichtyosis is very rare and is mainly to be differentiated from simple dry skin (xerosis) and from hereditary ichtyosis (autosomal dominant), that occurs usually before the age of 20.

Besides the neoplasia treatment, hydratation of the skin is helpful.

Dermatomyositis (Figures 8 and 9) can be idiopathic or cancer – associated (25% of the cases). It is a connective tissue disorder of unknown etiology, characterized by a lympho-plasmatocytic infiltration of skin and muscles, leading to atrophy and sclerosis. The disease usually appears very progressively but results finally in major motor impairment, due to muscle weakness.

Skin lesions usually start with periorbital heliotrop edematous skin rash and erythematous papules on the extensor surfaces of joints (Gottron's papules). Poikiloderma, peringueal teleangectasias and papular violaceous erythema over the involved skin are often present (forehead, cheeks, neck and upper chest).

The most commonly associated neoplasia with dermatomyosis are those of the female genital tract and respiratory tumors. Usually, tumor is diagnosed within one year of the dermatomyositis appearance, but the paraneoplastic syndrome can occur simultaneously or after the discovery of the neoplastic disease [12, 13].

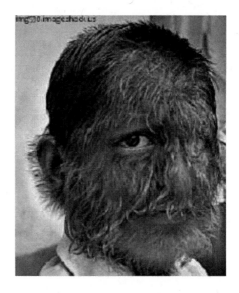

Figure 10. Hypertrichosis lanuginosa: excessive growth of fine, non pigmented hair.

In idiopathic cases, as in neoplasia – associated cases, corticoids and immunosuppressive drugs are usually effective. In neoplasia – associated cases, the course of dermatomyositis usually follows that of the tumor.

Hypertrichosis lanuginosa (Figure 10) consists in the sudden appearance of long, fine, non pigmented hair. Lanugo hairs initially involve face and ears but can eventually involve the whole hair bearing skin.

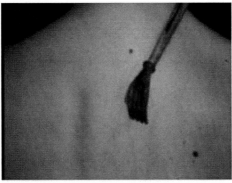

Figure 11. Pruritus: evidence of scratching and lichenification.

The syndrome is more common in women and usually occurs when tumor is already disseminated [14].

Hypertrichosis lanuginosa must be differentiated from hirsutism, characterized by excessive androgen-sensitive hair growth (thick hairs) distributed in adult male pattern, but also from acquired non paraneoplastic hypertrichosis that can be associated with a variety of drugs and morbid conditions. It has been suggested that hypertrichosis lanuginosa might be the consequence of cytoreductive chemotherapy;, this causal link is not clearly established in most cases.

Hypertrichosis lanuginosa is most commonly associated with adenocarcinomas of the lung and colon. It is also described in other solid tumors (pancreas, breast, kidney, gallbladder, bladder) as well as in leukemia and Ewing's sarcoma.

It may regress with appropriate associated cancer therapy. Cosmetic management includes shaving and depilation (mechanical and chemical).

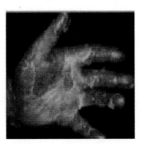

Figure 12. Exfoliative dermatitis: erythema and scaling, quite non specific.

Pruritus (Figure 11) may be the initial feature of an occult malignancy however it is usually a sign of advanced disease with poor prognosis. It is most frequently found in patients with Hodgkin's disease (it used to be a B symptom !) but is also common in polycythemia vera, cutaneous T cell lymphomas and other neoplasms.

Pruritus is a subjective perception and, in cases associated with cancer, the skin is usually xerotic or normal. However, severe pruritus quickly leads, to skin excoriations and subsequent scaring [15].

Failure to determine a dermatological cause to generalized pruritus necessitates evaluation for an underlying systemic disease (drug hypersensitivity, liver disease , ...) including cancer.

Emollient creams can be soothing, especially on irritated excoriated skin.

Exfoliative dermatitis (Figure 12) consists of a progressive erythema followed by scaling (hence its name) [16]. It is usually due to drug intolerance.

Cancer associated exfoliative dermatitis, represents less than 10% of the syndrome. It is then mainly associated with cutaneous Tcell lymphomas, other non Hodgkin's lymphomas and sometimes Hodgkin's disease.

Pachydermoperiostosis (Figure 13) is often associated with digital clubbing. Most often it is primary and and part of a familial inherited syndrome (Touraine − Solente − Golé syndrome) which is usually diagnosed early in life. Pachydermoperiostosis. is characterized by acromegalic features with thickening of the skin and creation of new folds, thickened lips, ears and lids. Macroglossia is often present as well as thickening of forehead and scalp.

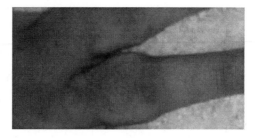

Figure 13. Pachydermoperiostosis (often associated with digital clubbing).

Isolated digital clubbing is a much more common paraneoplastic syndrome than pachydermoperiostosis.

Treatment of the associated cancer can improve periostosis but has little impact on clubbing.

Both are mainly associated with bronchogenic carcinomas [17].

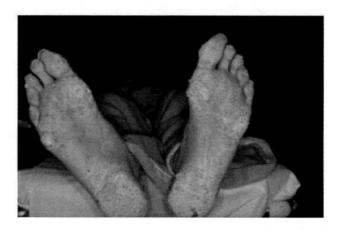

Figure 14. Hyperkeratosis (plantar).

Hyperkeratosis (Figure 14) consists of hyperkeratotic nodules on the skin; it can represent a paraneoplastic manifestation of cutaneous Tcell lymphomas.

It must be differentiated from disseminated squamous cell carcinomas or keratoacanthomas, lupus erythematosus, various infections and halogenodermatosis [18].

PARANEOPLASTIC SKIN MANIFESTATIONS CAUSED BY TUMOR-PRODUCED MECHANISM

Although it can be argued that such skin manifestations are not truly paraneoplastic, in the strict sense of the word, they are clearly associated with cancer without representing a metastatic spread.

These manifestations are important in terms of clinical diagnosis and their impact can be, occasionally, more important and more threatening than the cancer itself.

Table 3. Paraneoplastic skin manifestations specifically caused by a tumor-produced mecanism

Skin manifestation	Associated malignancy and putative cause
Melanosis	Melanoma producing melanin and\ or tumor with ectopic ACTH secretion.
Necrolytic migratory erythema	Glucagonoma producing glucagon or related products
Flushing (and pellagra)	Carcinoids (digestive tract, lung, ovary) producing serotonin
Amyloid deposits	Multiple myeloma and lymphoproliferative disorders producing paraproteins (light chains)
Weber Christian syndrome	Pancreatic cancer with lipase production (?)
Livedo reticularis and/or vaculitis	Lymphomas associated with cryoglobulinemia
Hirsutism	Adrenal and genital cancers with hyperandrogenism
Gynecomastia	Estrogen or HCG secreting tumors (germinal , adrenal and lung cancer)

They always follow a parallel course to that of the malignant tumor and most often disappears when the latter is controlled.

More importantly, their pathophysiological mechanism has been elucidated in most instances which often provides a possibility for symptomatic relief (Table 3).

Melanosis (Figure 15) is a diffuse grey to black skin pigmentation due to melanin deposits from a melanoma, accentuated on sun exposed areas, scars, nipples and skin folds (axilla, groins) [19]. At that stage, the tumor is often disseminated and presents with obvious metastases, especially in the liver. It is not uncommon, in such cases, that large amounts of melanin are excreted in the urine (melaninuria), making it look dark or even black when exposed to air for a while.

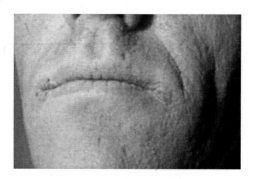

Figure 15. Melanosis: dark pigmentation due to melanin deposits.

Because ACTH has a structural similarity to the melanotropic hormone, ACTH secreting tumors (most often small cell lung carcinomas) can be responsible for a similar pigmentation (Figure 16), which resembles that seen in Addison's disease [20]. However, patients with paraneoplastic hypercorticism due to ectopic ACTH secretion by a tumor do not usually exhibit classical signs of Cushing's disease and, in most of them, skin pigmentation, edema and hypokalemia are the prominent clinical signs.

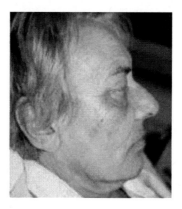

Figure 16. Addisonian's pigmentation due to ACTH secreting lung cancer.

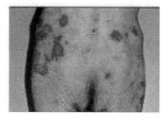

Figure 17. Necrolytic migratory erythema: blistering and epidermal necrosis.

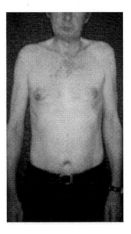

Figure 18. Flushing from carcinoid syndrome: end stage permanent vasodilatation.

Melanosis has to be further distinguished from other skin pigmentations (melanocytic and non melanocytic) due to medications (e.g. silver, arsenic), hemochromatosis, acanthosis nigricans and other less common conditions.

Necrolytic migratory erythema (Figure 17) is specifically associated with glucagonoma and thus, diabetes is a common associated feature, as well as diarrhea [21].

Skin manifestations consist of erythematous macules and papules that progress to blistering and epidermal necrosis. Lesions are typically located on pretibial area or periorificial area such as groin, anogenitalia including buttocks, as well as peribucal and perinasal. Lesions have a centrifugal extension.

Lesions usually clear after tumor resection but do persist in case of metastatic disease, in which case, somatostatin analogues can be benefical, as they suppress glucagon secretion and subsequent symptomatology. It is indeed probable that skin lesions are directly or indirectly related to glucagon overproduction by the tumor.

Flushing (Figure 18) consists of episodic reddening of the face and neck leading to chronic local vasodilatation, and namely to an erythematous, plethoric facies. Flushing is quite pathognomonic of the carcinoid syndrome, which is seen with serotonine secreting tumors.

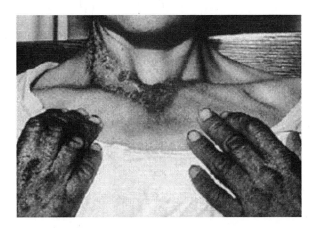

Figure 19. Pellagra-like syndrome associated with a carcinoid tumor.

These are mostly located in the terminal ileon and, since serotonine is destroyed in the liver, flushing only occurs in case of liver metastases. For the other serotonine-secreting tumors (ovary, lung, thyroid), there is no passage of the tumoral secretion through the liver, and flushing can therefore appear without liver metastases and at much earlier stages [22]. Dosage of urinary excretion of 5-HIAA is diagnostic and discriminates from other flushes, namely those related to mastocytosis.

Besides flushing and its cutaneous consequences, carcinoid syndrome consists of persistent diarrhea, peripheral edema, and in 20% of the cases – mainly patients with bronchial carcinoïds –of a sclerosis of the pulmonary valve, leading to tricuspid insufficiency and right cardiac failure [23].

Tryptophane is a precursor of serotonine, which is needed for the synthesis of niacin (vitamine PP). In patients with carcinoid syndrome, tryptophan can be derived for the synthesis of serotonine and a pellagra-like syndrome may appear: it consists of an erythemo-desquamative dermatitis (Figure 19) on sun-exposed areas, possibly with diarrhea and dementia.

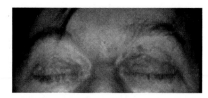

Figure 20. Amyloid deposit: waxy, yellow dermic plaques.

The carcinoid syndrome regresses completely if the liver metastases (in case of intestinal carcinoid) or the non ileal carcinoid are eradicated ; for inoperable disease, somatostatine and its derivatives can provide symptomatic relief for the flushing and the diarrhea. Cardiac surgery may be necessary in case of pulmonary valvular insufficiency.

Amyloid deposits (Figure 20): consists of waxy yellow or pink plaques and nodules on the skin in patients suffering from tumors associated with light chain gammapathies (multiple myeloma, Waldenström's macroglobulinemia, monoclonal gammapathy of unknown significance) or from primary AL amyloidosis. It can be associated with a typical periorbital purpura, most likely due to factor X deficiency, resulting from the binding of factor X to amyloid fibrils [24].

Besides the skin, other organs can be infiltrated by amyloid, namely the tongue (macroglossia) and the heart. The lungs and the digestive tract are also frequently involved in AL amyloidosis.

There is no specific treatment for AL amyloidosis associated with a neoplastic disease, besides control of the latter disease.

Weber Christian syndrome (Figure 21): consists of recurrent episodes of deep nodular lesions (nodular panniculitis), usually on the legs. The nodules are, inflammatory and painful, they progress to necrosis of the subcutaneous adipose tissue, with fistulisation [25]

It is a rare manifestation of various pancreatic diseases (namely chronic pancreatitis with cytosteatonecrosis) including pancreatic carcinoma.

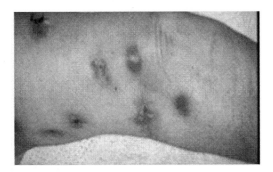

Figure 21. Weber Christian syndrome: subcutaneous fat necrosis.

Livedo reticularis and vasculitis (Figure 22) is rarely associated with cancer. Livedo reticularis consists of cyanotic, reddish-blue, mottled discolorations in a net-like pattern, that are increased by cold. Vasculitis (Figure 23) usually manifests as painful, palpable inflammatory purpuric nodules, that can undergo necrosis. The histologic examination is diagnostic [26].

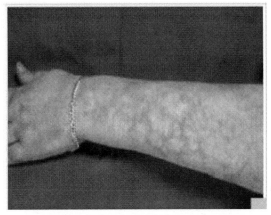

Figure 22. Livedo reticularis: cyanotic discoloration increased by cold exposure.

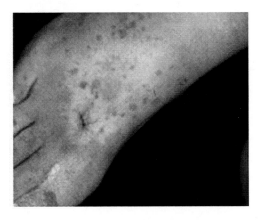

Figure 23. Vasculitis: palpable purpura evolving into hemorrhagic necrosis.

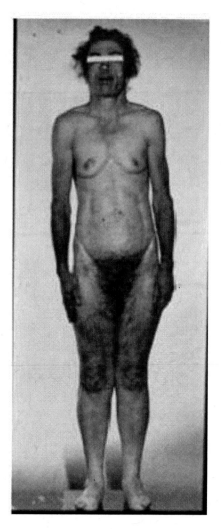

Figure 24. Hirsutism: excessive growth of hair in a masculine distribution.

These skin manifestations are typical of various forms of vasculopathies unrelated to cancer. However, they can be seen in association with some neoplastic diseases such as multiple myeloma, Waldenström's macroglobulinemia and lymphoproliferative disorders, mainly non Hodgkin's lymphomas [27]. In these cases, cryoglobulinemia is often present.

Hirsutism (Figure 24) is to be differentiated from hypertrichosis, namely hypertrichosis lanuginosa, that has been already discussed.

Morbid hirsutism is caused by excessive androgen secretion, usually from an adrenal or genital tumor. It is more difficult to recognize in males than in females, since it takes a typical masculine distribution.

In children such tumors can be associated with precocious and excessive puberty. In adults, excessive androgen secretion is associated with modified sexual behaviour and perturbed genital functions.

Various drugs can also be responsible for excessive growth of body hair, wether it causes hirsutism or hypertrichosis [28].

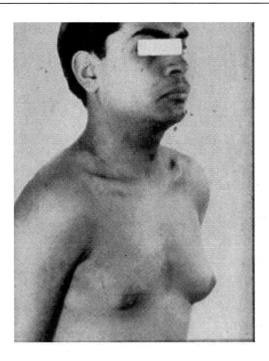

Figure 25. Gynecomastia.

Gynecomastia (Figure 25) can be associated with estrogen or HCG secreting tumors, although most cases are not associated with neoplasia [29].

Estrogens can be produced by testicular or adrenocortical tumors whether HCG secretion can be eutopic (germ cell tumors) or ectopic, mainly from bronchial, hepatocellular and renal carcinomas. Paraneoplastic gynecomastia usually runs a parallel course to that of the malignant tumor. Symptomatic therapy can consist of tamoxifen.

CONCLUSION

Skin can provide important clues for the recognition of many systemic diseases, namely cancer. This may be particularly important if the dermatologic manifestation precedes the overt signs and symptoms of the malignant disease and thus leads to early diagnosis. As the course of the cutaneous paraneoplastic disease may follow that of the malignancy, skin manifestations can sometimes mirror efficacy or failure of anticancer therapy.

Paraneoplastic skin syndromes are not frequent. In a prospective series [30], pruritus and xerosis were the commonest "paraneoplastic" dermatologic manifestations and occurred mainly in patients with hematological malignancies.

In true paraneoplastic syndromes, the mechanism linking them to the malignancy is usually unknown. In addition, since these skin manifestations can be seen in patients without cancer, the strength of the association with a malignancy is variable. Nevertheless, acrokeratosis paraneoplastica, hypertrichosis lanuginosa, erythema gyratum repens, hypertrophic osteoarthropathy, dermatomyositis and Sweet's syndrome are often – although not always – associated with a malignant tumor. Recognition of any of these potential paraneoplastic skin disorders should lead to a strong suspicion for an occult malignancy and trigger appropriate work-up. In case of negative investigation, a high suspicion level for an occult malignancy must be maintained for years.

Paraneoplastic skin manifestations with well known pathophysiological mechanisms related to a tumor, such as cutaneous amyloidosis, melanic pigmentation, vasculitis, carcinoid flushing, hirsutism, gynecomastia and others, can be responsible for signs and symptoms requiring specific therapies. These manifestations usually follow a course that is clearly related to that of the tumor and can thus serve as surrogates for its evolution.

It is hoped that the recognition of these paraneoplastic skin disorders may contribute to an earlier diagnosis of malignancy and trigger research for a better understanding of their mecanisms, potentially leading to novel therapies.

The figures have been adapted from their original file, and the authors of this chapter thank their different sources for this.

REFERENCES

[1]   Cohen PR, Kurzrock R: Mucocutaneous paraneoplastic syndromes. *Semin Oncol.1997*;24:334-359.

[2]   Pipkin CA, Lio PA: Cutaneous manifestations of internal malignancies: an overview.*Dermatol Clin.* 2008;26:31-43.

[3]   Kaminska-Winciorek G, Brzezinska-Weislo L, Lis-Swiety A et al: Paraneoplastic type of acanthosis nigricans in patient with hepatocellular carcinoma. *Adv Med Sci.* 2007; 52:254-256.

[4]   Kaoulaouzidis A, Leiper K: Tripe palms or acanthosis palmaris. *Intern Med J.*2007;37:502.

[5]   Wieland CN, Kumar N: Sign of Leser-Trelat. *Int J Dermatol.* 2008;47:643-644.

[6]   Poligone B, Christensen SR, Lazova R et al: Bazex syndrome (acrokeratosis paraneoplastica). *Lancet.*2007;369:530.

[7]   Lin W, Lin WC, Chiu CS et al.:Paraneoplastic Sweet's syndrome in a patient with hemophagocytic syndrome.*Int J Dermatol.*2008;47:305-307.

[8]   Cohen PR: Sweet's syndrome-a comprehensive review of an acute febrile neutrophilic dermatosis.*Orphanet J Rare Dis.*2007;2:34.

[9]   Jacob SE, Weisman RS, Kerdel FA: Pyoderma gangrenosum-rebel without a cure ? *Int J Dermatol.*2008;47:192-194.

[10]   Ravié-Nikolié A, Milicié V, Jovovic-Dagovic B et al.: Gyrate erythema associated with metastatic tumor of gastrointestinal tract. *Dermatol Online J.*2006;12:11.

[11]   Mazereeuw J, Bonafé JL: Xerosis. *Ann Dermatol Venereol.*2002;129:137-142.

[12]   Harrison BA, Heck SI, Hood AF: A fatal case of dermatomyositis with underlying metastatic esophageal adenocarcinoma. *Cutis.*2008;81:26-28.

[13]   Kikuchi K, Seto Y, Matsubara T et al.: Amyopathic dermatomyositis associated with esophageal cancer. *Int J Dermatol.*2008;47:310-311.

[14]   Farina MC, Tarin N, Grilli R et al.: Acquired hypertrichosis lanuginosa: report and review of the literature. *J Surg Oncol.* 1998;68:199-203.

[15]   Stadie V, Marsch WC: Itching attacks with generalized hyperhydrosis as initial symptoms of Hodgkin's disease. *J Europ Acad Dermatol Venereol.*2003;17:559-561.

[16]   Zhu X, Zhang B: Paraneoplastic pemphigus : *J Dermatol.*2007;34:503-511.

[17] Ikeda F, Okada H, Mizuno M et al.: Pachydermoperiostosis associated with juvenile polyps of the stomach and gastric andenocarcinoma. *J Gastroenterol.*2004;39:470-474.

[18] Resnik KS, Di Leonardo M: Incidental granular parakeratotic cornification in carcinomas.*Am J Dermatophath.*2007;29:264-269.

[19] PauloFilho T, Trinidate Neto PB, Reis JC et al.: Diffuse cutaneous melanosis in malignant melanoma. *Dermatol Online J.*2007;13:9.

[20] Noorlander I, Elte JW, Nanintveld OC et al.: A case of recurrent non small cell lung cancer and paraneoplastic Cushing's syndrome. *Lung cancer.*2006;51:251-255.

[21] Chaw L, Krop TM, Hood AF: What is your diagnosis? Necrolytic migratory erythema associated with a glucagonoma. *Cutis.*2008;25:30-32.

[22] Bofek A, Rachowska R, Rajewska J et al.: Carcinoid syndrome with angioedema and urticaria. *Arch Dermato.*2008;144:691-692.

[23] Castillo JG, Filsoufi F, Rahmanian PB et al.: Early and late results of valvular surgery for carcinoid heart disease. *J Am Coll Cardiol.*2008;51:1507-1509.

[24] Gül V, Soylu S, Kilic A et al.: Monoclonal gammapathy of undetermined significance diagnosed by cutaneous manifestations of AL amyloidosis. *Europ J Dermatol.*2007;17:255-256.

[25] Weening RH, Mehrany K: Dermal and pannicular manifestations of internal malignancy. *Dermatol Clin.*2008;26:31-43.

[26] Simon Z, Tarr T, Tom L et al.: Cutaneous vasculitis as an initiating paraneoplastic symptom in Hodgkin lymphoma. *Rheumatol Int.*2008;7:719-723.

[27] El Tal AK, Tamous Z: Cutaneous vascular disorders associated with internal malignancy.*Dermatol Clin.*2008;26:45-57.

[28] Wendelin D, Pope D, Mallory S: Hypertrichosis. *J Am Acad Dermatol.* 2003;48:161-179.

[29] Braunstein GD: Gynecomastia. *N Engl J Med* 2007;357:1229-1237.

[30] Kilic A, Gul U, Soylu S: Skin findings in internal malignant diseases. *Intern J Dermatol.* 2007;46:1055-1060.

In: Handbook of Skin Care in Cancer Patients
Editors: Pierre Vereecken and Ahmad Awada

ISBN: 978-1-61668-419-8
© 2012 Nova Science Publishers, Inc.

Chapter 15

TATTOOS AND CAMOUFLAGE: NOT TO FORGET!

Dachelet Claire[1], Titeca Géraldine[2], Comas Marine[3], Steels Emmanuelle[4] and Vereecken Pierre[5]

[1]Cliniques Universitaires Saint-Luc –Mont-Godinne, Belgium
[2]Hôpital Notre-Dame, Gosselies, Belgium
[3]CHIREC and Erasme Hospital, Brussels, Belgium
[4]CHU-Brugmann and Chirec, Brussels, Belgium
[5]Cliniques Universitaires Saint-Luc, Brussels, Belgium

Cosmetic skin care including tattoos and camouflages is an important issue in cancer patients, and these techniques have to be considered as a powerful help in many patients.

The medical tattoo allows the aesthetic repair of some areas of the body and quite specifically lips and breast, and eyelids. This is obtained thanks to the use of pigments of iron oxide with a wide choice of colors.

After a local anaesthesia, the dermatologist chooses a complexion which will be as close as possible to the color of the skin of the patient (Figure 1a and b). There are some side effects according to the choice and the size of the pigments which are used. Depigmentation can also be realized with different kind of lasers.

The tattoo and the permanent make-up are mainly used to re-pigment the areolas of the women after surgery for a breast cancer (surgical ablation). This represents the "end" of the therapeutic course and the resumption of a normal life. The scars of the breast are not always beautiful since these are located in the connection area between an elastic tissue (areola) and a not elastic tissue (skin of the breast). This emphasizes the importance to offer aesthetic procedures such as medical tattoos (Figure 1c).

The repigmentation consists to introduce into the dermis , insoluble colored particles. The palette of the available pigments is wide and it is possible to reproduce precisely the natural color of the skin. These pigments are stable. They are the object of an approval according to medico – surgical norms.

The session of dermopigmentation is refunded by the Medical Insurance in Belgium. The session time is approximately 45 minutes and a single intervention is in most cases enough.

New generation pigments clear up, but does not disappear. This treatment can be however repeated after three years.

These techniques are also used in the case of scars of the face (labiopalatine clefts, accidents, burns). According to the area, the effect is not always perfect, but contributes to improve the aesthetics. In some cases, the tattoo gives better results, in the others, the make-up is more successful.

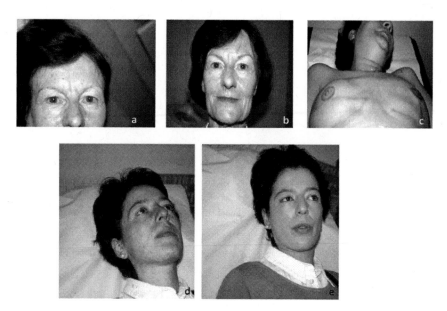

Figure 1. Tattoos and camouflage in patients.

It is a technique which helps to become reconciled with her (or his) own body.

Camouflaging skin lesions is a technique of makeup with special, non comedogenic, hypoallergenic, waterproof creams and with covering power. A lot of medical problems with cosmetic consequences can unfortunately not be treated effectively by medical treatments ; the correct use of camouflage can help efficiently oncology patients and improve there quality of life and there appearance.

This make-up is made by means of specific compact creams, different from other daily use products. Basically, they are subtypes of make-up and they consist of various coloring agents in an oily or not oily base. They are non-comedogenic, hypoallergenic, waterproof and have an important covering power.

This camouflage can be used to correct pale cutaneous zones. Camouflage is also used to hide red lesions like angioma, telangiectasia or to correct hyperpigmented lesions like scars.

The aim of camouflage is to correct, compensate for excesses, to unify the complexion (Figure 1 d and e).

It is important to teach the patient to transform a defect and then to work on the integration of this modification. Beside this, a light make-up has to be proposed to the patient in order to give a blow of brightness. Perfect color match is impossible but the use of different colours can surely bring the most natural effect.

Appendix 1. Common Terminology Criteria for Adverse Events (CTCAE) Version 4.02 (Adapted from U.S. Department of Health and Human Services, National Institutes of Health, National Cancer Institute

The NCI Common Terminology Criteria for Adverse Events is a descriptive terminology which can be utilized for Adverse Events (AE) reporting. A grading (severity) scale is provided for each AE term.

Grade refers to the severity of the AE, from grade 1 (mild) to grade 5 (death related to AE). A single dash (-) indicates a grade is not available.

Grade 1:   Mild; asymptomatic or mild symptoms; clinical or diagnostic observations only; intervention not indicated.

Grade 2:   Moderate; minimal, local or non-invasive intervention indicated; limiting age –appropriate instrumental activities of daily living (ADL)

Grade 3:   Severe or medically significant but not immediately life-threatening; hospitalization or prolongation of hospitalization indicated; disabling; limiting self care ADL

Grade 4:   life-threatening consequences; urgent intervention indicated.

Grade 5:   Death related to AE

Appendix 1. Table

MedDRA v12.0 Code	CTCAE v4.0 SOC	CTCAE v4.0 Term	Grade 1	Grade 2	Grade 3	Grade 4	Grade 5	CTCAE v4.0 AE Term Definition
10001760	Skin and subcutaneous tissue disorders	Alopecia	Hair loss of up to 50% of normal for that individual that is not obvious from a distance but only on close inspection; a different hair style may be required to cover the hair loss but it does not require a wig or hair piece to camouflage	Hair loss of >50% normal for that individual that is readily apparent to others; a wig or hair piece is necessary if the patient desires to completely camouflage the hair loss; associated with psychosocial impact	-	-	-	A disorder characterized by a decrease in density of hair compared to normal for a given individual at a given age and body location.
10005901	Skin and subcutaneous tissue disorders	Body odor	Mild odor; physician intervention not indicated; self care interventions	Pronounced odor; psychosocial impact; patient seeks medical intervention	-	-	-	A disorder characterized by an abnormal body smell resulting from the growth of bacteria on the body.
10006556	Skin and subcutaneous tissue disorders	Bullous dermatitis	Asymptomatic; blisters covering <10% BSA	Blisters covering 10 - 30% BSA; painful blisters; limiting instrumental ADL	Blisters covering >30% BSA; limiting self care ADL	Blisters covering >30% BSA; associated with fluid or electrolyte abnormalities; ICU care or burn unit indicated	Death	A disorder characterized by inflammation of the skin characterized by the presence of bullae which are filled with fluid.
10013786	Skin and subcutaneous tissue disorders	Dry skin	Covering <10% BSA and no associated erythema or pruritus	Covering 10 - 30% BSA and associated with erythema or pruritus; limiting instrumental ADL	Covering >30% BSA and associated with pruritus; limiting self care ADL	-	-	A disorder characterized by flaky and dull skin; the pores are generally fine, the texture is a papery thin texture.

MedDRA v12.0 Code	CTCAE v4.0 SOC	Term	Grade 1	Grade 2	Grade 3	Grade 4	Grade 5	Term Definition
10015218	Skin and subcutaneous tissue disorders	Erythema multiforme	Target lesions covering <10% BSA and not associated with skin tenderness	Target lesions covering 10 - 30% BSA and associated with skin tenderness	Target lesions covering >30% BSA and associated with oral or genital erosions	Target lesions covering >30% BSA; associated with fluid or electrolyte abnormalities; ICU care or burn unit indicated	Death	A disorder characterized by target lesions (a pink-red ring around a pale center).
10015277	Skin and subcutaneous tissue disorders	Erythroderma	-	Erythema covering >90% BSA without associated symptoms; limiting instrumental ADL	Erythema covering >90% BSA with associated symptoms (e.g., pruritus or tenderness); limiting self care ADL	Erythema covering >90% BSA with associated fluid or electrolyte abnormalities; ICU care or burn unit indicated	Death	A disorder characterized by generalized inflammatory erythema and exfoliation. The inflammatory process involves > 90% of the body surface area.
10016241	Skin and subcutaneous tissue disorders	Fat atrophy	Covering <10% BSA and asymptomatic	Covering 10 - 30% BSA and associated with erythema or tenderness; limiting instrumental ADL	Covering >30% BSA; associated with erythema or tenderness; limiting self-care ADL	-	-	A disorder characterized by shrinking of adipose tissue.
10020112	Skin and subcutaneous tissue disorders	Hirsutism	In women, increase in length, thickness or density of hair in a male distribution that the patient is able to camouflage by periodic shaving, bleaching, or removal of hair	In women, increase in length, thickness or density of hair in a male distribution that requires daily shaving or consistent destructive means of hair removal to camouflage; associated with psychosocial impact	-	-	-	A disorder characterized by the presence of excess hair growth in women in anatomic sites where growth is considered to be a secondary male characteristic and under androgen control (beard, moustache, chest, abdomen).

Appendix 1. Table (continued)

MedDRA v12.0 Code	CTCAE v4.0 SOC	CTCAE v4.0 Term	Grade 1	Grade 2	Grade 3	Grade 4	Grade 5	CTCAE v4.0 AE Term Definition
10020642	Skin and subcutaneous tissue disorders	Hyperhidrosis	Limited to one site (palms, soles, or axillae); self care interventions	Involving >1 site; patient seeks medical intervention; associated with psychosocial impact	Generalized involving sites other than palms, soles, or axillae; associated with electrolyte/hemodynamic imbalance	-	-	A disorder characterized by excessive perspiration.
10020864	Skin and subcutaneous tissue disorders	Hypertrichosis	Increase in length, thickness or density of hair that the patient is either able to camouflage by periodic shaving or removal of hairs or is not concerned enough about the overgrowth to use any form of hair removal	Increase in length, thickness or density of hair at least on the usual exposed areas of the body [face (not limited to beard/moustache area) plus/minus arms] that requires frequent shaving or use of destructive means of hair removal to camouflage; associated with psychosocial impact	-	-	-	A disorder characterized by hair density or length beyond the accepted limits of normal in a particular body region, for a particular age or race.
10021013	Skin and subcutaneous tissue disorders	Hypohidrosis	-	Symptomatic; limiting instrumental ADL	Increase in body temperature; limiting self care ADL	Heat stroke	Death	A disorder characterized by reduced sweating.
10062315	Skin and subcutaneous tissue disorders	Lipohypertrophy	Asymptomatic and covering <10% BSA	Covering 10 - 30% BSA and associated tenderness; limiting instrumental ADL	Covering >30% BSA and associated tenderness and narcotics or NSAIDs indicated; lipohypertrophy; limiting self care ADL	-	-	A disorder characterized by hypertrophy of the subcutaneous adipose tissue at the site of multiple subcutaneous injections of insulin.

MedDRA v12.0 Code	SOC	CTCAE v4.0 Term	Grade 1	Grade 2	Grade 3	Grade 4	Grade 5	Term Definition
10028691	Skin and subcutaneous tissue disorders	Nail discoloration	Asymptomatic; clinical or diagnostic observations only; intervention not indicated		-	-	-	A disorder characterized by a change in the color of the nail plate.
10049281	Skin and subcutaneous tissue disorders	Nail loss	Asymptomatic separation of the nail bed from the nail plate or nail loss	Symptomatic separation of the nail bed from the nail plate or nail loss; limiting instrumental ADL	-	-	-	A disorder characterized by loss of all or a portion of the nail.
10062283	Skin and subcutaneous tissue disorders	Nail ridging	Asymptomatic; clinical or diagnostic observations only; intervention not indicated	-	-	-	-	A disorder characterized by vertical or horizontal ridges on the nails.
10033474	Skin and subcutaneous tissue disorders	Pain of skin	Mild pain	Moderate pain; limiting instrumental ADL	Severe pain; limiting self care ADL	-	-	A disorder characterized by marked discomfort sensation in the skin.
10054524	Skin and subcutaneous tissue disorders	Palmar-plantar erythrodysesthesia syndrome	Minimal skin changes or dermatitis (e.g., erythema, edema, or hyperkeratosis) without pain	Skin changes (e.g., peeling, blisters, bleeding, edema, or hyperkeratosis) with pain; limiting instrumental ADL	Severe skin changes (e.g., peeling, blisters, bleeding, edema, or hyperkeratosis) with pain; limiting self care ADL	-	-	A disorder characterized by redness, marked discomfort, swelling, and tingling in the palms of the hands or the soles of the feet.
10054541	Skin and subcutaneous tissue disorders	Periorbital edema	Soft or non-pitting	Indurated or pitting edema; topical intervention indicated	Edema associated with visual disturbance; increased intraocular pressure, glaucoma or retinal	-	-	A disorder characterized by swelling due to an excessive accumulation of fluid around the orbits of the face.

Appendix 1. Table (continued)

MedDRA v12.0 Code	CTCAE v4.0 SOC	CTCAE v4.0 Term	Grade 1	Grade 2	Grade 3	Grade 4	Grade 5	CTCAE v4.0 AE Term Definition
					hemorrhage; optic neuritis; diuretics indicated; operative intervention indicated			
10034966	Skin and subcutaneous tissue disorders	Photosensitivity	Painless erythema and erythema covering <10% BSA	Tender erythema covering 10 - 30% BSA	Erythema covering >30% BSA and erythema with blistering; photosensitivity; oral corticosteroid therapy indicated; pain control indicated (e.g., narcotics or NSAIDs)	Life-threatening consequences; urgent intervention indicated	Death	A disorder characterized by an increase in sensitivity of the skin to light.
10037087	Skin and subcutaneous tissue disorders	Pruritus	Mild or localized; topical intervention indicated	Intense or widespread; intermittent; skin changes from scratching (e.g., edema, papulation, excoriations, lichenification, oozing/crusts); oral intervention indicated; limiting instrumental ADL	Intense or widespread; constant; limiting self care ADL or sleep; oral corticosteroid or immunosuppressive therapy indicated	-	-	A disorder characterized by an intense itching sensation.
10037549	Skin and subcutaneous tissue disorders	Purpura	Combined area of lesions covering <10% BSA	Combined area of lesions covering 10 - 30% BSA; bleeding with trauma	Combined area of lesions covering >30% BSA; spontaneous bleeding	-	-	A disorder characterized by hemorrhagic areas of the skin and mucous membrane. Newer lesions appear reddish in color. Older lesions are usually a darker

MedDRA v12.0 Code	CTCAE v4.0 SOC	CTCAE v4.0 Term	Grade 1	Grade 2	Grade 3	Grade 4	Grade 5	Term Definition
								purple color and eventually become a brownish-yellow color.
10037847	Skin and subcutaneous tissue disorders	Rash acneiform	Papules and/or pustules covering <10% BSA, which may or may not be associated with symptoms of pruritus or tenderness	Papules and/or pustules covering 10 - 30% BSA, which may or may not be associated with symptoms of pruritus or tenderness; associated with psychosocial impact; limiting instrumental ADL	Papules and/or pustules covering >30% BSA, which may or may not be associated with symptoms of pruritus or tenderness; limiting self care ADL; associated with local superinfection with oral antibiotics indicated	Papules and/or pustules covering any % BSA, which may or may not be associated with symptoms of pruritus or tenderness and are associated with extensive superinfection with IV antibiotics indicated; life-threatening consequences	Death	A disorder characterized by an eruption of papules and pustules, typically appearing in face, scalp, upper chest and back.
10037868	Skin and subcutaneous tissue disorders	Rash maculo-papular	Macules/papules covering <10% BSA with or without symptoms (e.g., pruritus, burning, tightness)	Macules/papules covering 10 - 30% BSA with or without symptoms (e.g., pruritus, burning, tightness); limiting instrumental ADL	Macules/papules covering >30% BSA with or without associated symptoms; limiting self care ADL	-	-	A disorder characterized by the presence of macules (flat) and papules (elevated). Also known as morbilliform rash, it is one of the most common cutaneous adverse events, frequently affecting the upper trunk, spreading centripetally and associated with pruritis.

Appendix 1. Table (continued)

MedDRA v12.0 Code	CTCAE v4.0 SOC	CTCAE v4.0 Term	Grade 1	Grade 2	Grade 3	Grade 4	Grade 5	CTCAE v4.0 AE Term Definition
10049120	Skin and subcutaneous tissue disorders	Scalp pain	Mild pain	Moderate pain; limiting instrumental ADL	Severe pain; limiting self care ADL	-	-	A disorder characterized by marked discomfort sensation in the skin covering the top and the back of the head.
10040799	Skin and subcutaneous tissue disorders	Skin atrophy	Covering <10% BSA; associated with telangiectasias or changes in skin color	Covering 10 - 30% BSA; associated with striae or adnexal structure loss	Covering >30% BSA; associated with ulceration	-	-	A disorder characterized by the degeneration and thinning of the epidermis and dermis.
10040865	Skin and subcutaneous tissue disorders	Skin hyperpigmentation	Hyperpigmentation covering <10% BSA; no psychosocial impact	Hyperpigmentation covering >10% BSA; associated psychosocial impact	-	-	-	A disorder characterized by darkening of the skin due to excessive melanin deposition.
10040868	Skin and subcutaneous tissue disorders	Skin hypopigmentation	Hypopigmentation or depigmentation covering <10% BSA; no psychosocial impact	Hypopigmentation or depigmentation covering >10% BSA; associated psychosocial impact	-	-	-	A disorder characterized by loss of skin pigment.
10051837	Skin and subcutaneous tissue disorders	Skin induration	Mild induration, able to move skin parallel to plane (sliding) and perpendicular to skin (pinching up)	Moderate induration, able to slide skin, unable to pinch skin; limiting instrumental ADL	Severe induration, unable to slide or pinch skin; limiting joint movement or orifice (e.g., mouth, anus); limiting self care ADL	Generalized; associated with signs or symptoms of impaired breathing or feeding	Death	A disorder characterized by an area of hardness in the skin.
10040947	Skin and subcutaneous tissue disorders	Skin ulceration	Combined area of ulcers <1 cm; nonblanchable erythema of intact skin with associated	Combined area of ulcers 1 - 2 cm; partial thickness skin loss involving skin or subcutaneous fat	Combined area of ulcers >2 cm; full-thickness skin loss involving damage to or necrosis of	Any size ulcer with extensive destruction, tissue necrosis, or damage to muscle,	Death	A disorder characterized by circumscribed, inflammatory and necrotic erosive

MedDRA v12.0 Code	CTCAE v4.0 SOC	CTCAE v4.0 Term	Grade 1	Grade 2	Grade 3	Grade 4	Grade 5	CTCAE v4.0 AE Term Definition
			warmth or edema		subcutaneous tissue that may extend down to fascia	bone, or supporting structures with or without full thickness skin loss		lesion on the skin.
10042033	Skin and subcutaneous tissue disorders	Stevens-Johnson syndrome			Skin sloughing covering <10% BSA with associated signs (e.g., erythema, purpura, epidermal detachment and mucous membrane detachment)	Skin sloughing covering 10 - 30% BSA with associated signs (e.g., erythema, purpura, epidermal detachment and mucous membrane detachment)	Death	A disorder characterized by less than 10% total body skin area separation of dermis. The syndrome is thought to be a hypersensitivity complex affecting the skin and the mucous membranes.
10043189	Skin and subcutaneous tissue disorders	Telangiectasia	Telangiectasias covering <10% BSA	Telangiectasias covering >10% BSA; associated with psychosocial impact	-	-	-	A disorder characterized by local dilatation of small vessels resulting in red discoloration of the skin or mucous membranes.
10044223	Skin and subcutaneous tissue disorders	Toxic epidermal necrolysis	-	-	-	Skin sloughing covering >=30% BSA with associated symptoms (e.g., erythema, purpura, or epidermal detachment)	Death	A disorder characterized by greater than 30% total body skin area separation of dermis. The syndrome is thought to be a hypersensitivity complex affecting the skin and the mucous membranes.

Appendix 1. Table (continued)

MedDRA v12.0 Code	CTCAE v4.0 SOC	CTCAE v4.0 Term	Grade 1	Grade 2	Grade 3	Grade 4	Grade 5	CTCAE v4.0 AE Term Definition
10046735	Skin and subcutaneous tissue disorders	Urticaria	Urticarial lesions covering <10% BSA; topical intervention indicated	Urticarial lesions covering 10 - 30% BSA; oral intervention indicated	Urticarial lesions covering >30% BSA; IV intervention indicated	-	-	A disorder characterized by an itchy skin eruption characterized by wheals with pale interiors and well-defined red margins.
10040785	Skin and subcutaneous tissue disorders	Skin and subcutaneous tissue disorders - Other, specify	Asymptomatic or mild symptoms; clinical or diagnostic observations only; intervention not indicated	Moderate; minimal, local or noninvasive intervention indicated; limiting age-appropriate instrumental ADL	Severe or medically significant but not immediately life-threatening; hospitalization or prolongation of existing hospitalization indicated; disabling; limiting self care ADL	Life-threatening consequences; urgent intervention indicated	Death	-

Comment: Instrumental ADL refer to preparing meals, shopping for groceries or clothes, using the thelephone, managing money,… and self care ADL refer to bathing, dressing and undressing, feeding self, using the toilet, taking medications, and not bedridden.

INDEX

#

20th century, 63

A

abuse, 12
access, 84, 149, 154, 159, 160, 161
accounting, 106, 110, 167
acid, 13, 14, 17, 83, 122, 137, 157
acne, 12, 18, 19, 90, 93, 124, 126, 142
acneiform eruption, vii, 9, 10, 11, 12, 13, 14, 15, 16, 17, 44, 72
Acrokeratosis paraneoplastic, x, 163, 166
ACTH, 173, 174
actinic keratosis, 65, 69
acute myelogenous leukemia, 167
adalimumab, 168
adenocarcinoma, 103, 107, 109, 110, 112, 114, 115, 180
adenopathy, 101
adipose, 176, 187, 188
adipose tissue, 176, 187, 188
adjustment, 4, 13, 16, 17
adult T-cell, 104
adults, 2, 80, 142, 178
adverse effects, 6, 18, 26, 29, 38, 87
adverse event, 25, 33, 36, 37, 42, 47, 67, 68, 69, 71, 72, 161, 191
aerodigestive tract, 102, 112
aerosols, 117
aesthetic, vii, x, 183
aesthetics, 184
age, 80, 141, 142, 145, 146, 152, 170, 185, 186, 188, 194
agonist, 34

alkaloids, 25, 63, 65, 70, 122, 150, 155, 156, 157, 159, 162
alkylation, 157
allergic reaction, 67
allergy, 12, 53, 58
alopecia, viii, 21, 22, 23, 24, 25, 26, 27, 28, 29, 30, 31, 32, 33, 34, 38, 45, 64, 67, 68, 69, 70, 71, 73, 98, 100, 103, 106, 109, 113
alopecia areata, 24, 27, 38, 100, 109, 113
alopecia ensue, viii, 21
alpha interferon, 33
alters, 36
amyloidosis, x, 163, 176, 180, 181
anaphylactic reactions, 64
anaphylaxis, 27, 67
anastomosis, 133, 136
anatomic site, 187
anatomy, 4, 37, 125
androgen, 30, 171, 178, 187
androgens, 122
angioedema, 181
angiogenesis, 3, 43
angioma, 124, 126, 184
anti-angiogenic agents, 72
antibiotic, 13, 15, 69, 86
antibody, 13, 18, 49, 92, 168
anti-cancer, 3, 10, 64
anticancer activity, 46
anticancer drug, 37, 159
antihistamines, 155, 156
anti-inflammatory drugs, 14, 55
antiseptic mouthwash, 15
antiseptic soaks, vii, 9
antitumor, 7, 69, 77, 150, 162
antitumor agent, 162
antiviral drugs, 13, 14
anus, 192
apoptosis, 3, 23, 25

arabinoside, 31, 34, 74
arginine, 85
argon, 145, 148
arrest, 24, 29
arrests, 23
arsenic, 61, 175
arterioles, 80
arteritis, 67
aspirate, 155
aspiration, 86, 101, 157
assessment, 7, 31, 33, 80, 85, 87, 119, 137
asymptomatic, 10, 185, 187
atrial myxoma, 109
atrophy, 4, 12, 65, 145, 158, 170, 187, 192
attachment, 22
authorities, 80, 119, 123, 124, 154
autonomy, viii, 79, 80
autopsy, 112
autosomal dominant, 170
awareness, 149
axilla, 101, 104, 164, 173

blood vessels, 152
bloodstream, 132
body image, 132
body mass index, 85
body weight, 85
bone, 67, 68, 69, 70, 81, 85, 158, 193
bone marrow, 67, 68, 69, 70, 158
brachytherapy, x, 75, 139, 142, 145
Braden Scale, viii, 79, 80
brain, 24, 109
brain tumor, 109
breakdown, 146
breast cancer, 7, 10, 28, 31, 34, 49, 60, 61, 69, 70,
    72, 75, 97, 98, 99, 100, 101, 106, 110, 133, 138,
    141, 142, 157, 183
breast carcinoma, 100, 101, 113
breathing, 192
brittle hair, 24
brittleness, 38, 39, 44, 45
burn, 53, 55, 101, 112, 143, 186, 187

B

bacteria, 3, 69, 90, 122, 130, 137, 186
bacterial infection, 85
bacterium, 29
basal cell carcinoma, 51, 52, 57, 100, 110, 141, 147
basal layer, 90
base, 70, 131, 184
base pair, 70
basement membrane, 4, 167
baths, 4, 126
Belgium, 9, 21, 28, 35, 63, 89, 95, 117, 119, 125,
    129, 139, 149, 163, 183
benefits, 13
benign, ix, 95, 103, 115, 141, 164, 166
benign skin lesions, ix, 95
beta-carotene, 57
bicarbonate, 156
bile, 115
bile duct, 115
biliary tract, 165
biologic therapy drugs, vii, 1
biopsy, 86, 90, 98, 106, 110, 133, 137, 138, 158
biosynthesis, 60
biotin, 45, 49
bladder cancer, 67, 69, 107, 165
bleaching, 187
bleeding, 72, 108, 189, 190
blepharitis, 15, 16
blood, 29, 80, 97, 121, 130, 133, 152, 153, 154, 155
blood flow, 29, 80, 133, 155

C

C reactive protein, 85
caffeine, 121, 122
calcifications, 110
calorie, 85
cancer, vii, viii, ix, x, 1, 3, 18, 21, 24, 25, 26, 27, 29,
    30, 33, 34, 37, 38, 40, 47, 48, 49, 51, 53, 58, 59,
    60, 63, 64, 67, 68, 70, 71, 73, 74, 76, 77, 80, 92,
    93, 95, 96, 97, 98, 99, 101, 103, 105, 106, 108,
    109, 110, 111, 112, 115, 129, 130, 131, 132, 133,
    135, 137, 138, 139, 147, 149, 152, 154, 159, 160,
    163, 164, 165, 167, 170, 171, 172, 173, 177, 178,
    179, 181, 183
cancer cells, 130
cancer patients, vii, 17, 21
cancer progression, 26
candidates, 85
capillary, 80, 130
carbon, 148
carbon dioxide, 148
carcinogenesis, 57, 142, 159
carcinoid syndrome, 175, 176
carcinoid tumor, 108, 114, 175
carcinoma, 3, 28, 52, 53, 67, 73, 76, 89, 96, 98, 99,
    100, 101, 102, 103, 106, 107, 108, 110, 111, 112,
    113, 114, 115, 137, 141, 152, 176
cardiomyopathy, 157
carotene, 57
carotenoids, 57
case studies, 106
catabolism, 68, 69

catheter, 145, 152, 153, 158, 159
Caucasian population, 126
CDK inhibitor, 90
CEE, 119, 122, 123, 124, 125
cell cycle, 43, 66
cell death, 150
cell division, 63, 70
cellulitis, 76, 131
cephalosporin, 13
cervical cancer, 67, 71
cervix, 32, 53, 96, 103, 109, 112, 137
chemical, 22, 29, 58, 66, 106, 117, 121, 124, 171
chemical bonds, 66
chemical characteristics, 121
chemotherapeutic agent, 1, 3, 25, 38, 55, 64, 70, 75, 160, 161
chemotherapy, vii, viii, x, 1, 2, 3, 5, 7, 18, 25, 27, 28, 30, 31, 32, 34, 35, 36, 38, 40, 41, 42, 43, 45, 47, 48, 49, 52, 55, 58, 59, 60, 61, 63, 64, 66, 67, 70, 72, 73, 74, 75, 135, 149, 152, 153, 154, 158, 159, 160, 161, 162, 171
childhood, 52, 57, 60, 147
children, 2, 47, 52, 104, 113, 178
chloasma, 126
cholecalciferol, 59
chondrosarcoma, 107
chromosome, 76
chronic lymphocytic leukemia, 104
chronic myelogenous, 60
chronobiology, 30
circulation, 97, 121, 133
classification, 3, 10, 36, 81, 82, 119, 131
class-specific side effects, vii, 9, 10
cleaning, 45, 83, 120
clinical diagnosis, 141, 173
clinical presentation, vii, 1, 29, 36, 47, 48, 103, 107, 110, 164
clinical symptoms, ix, 89
clinical trials, 76, 158, 159
closure, 85, 158
clothing, 57, 62
clubbing, 172
clusters, 161
coal, 122
coal tar, 122
coffee, 121
cognitive dysfunction, 152
cold compress, 5, 11
collaboration, 11, 154, 159
collagen, ix, 139, 140, 141
collateral, 133
colon, ix, 52, 67, 71, 95, 97, 100, 102, 106, 109, 110, 165, 171

colon cancer, 71, 106
colonization, 85
color, 14, 26, 103, 104, 105, 146, 183, 184, 189, 190, 191, 192
colorectal cancer, 7, 10, 15, 16, 18, 72, 74, 76, 92, 93, 110
commercial, 118
communication, 11
community, 59
compensation, 125
complications, 3, 4, 15, 18, 64, 75, 133, 138, 146, 149, 153
composition, 22, 58, 119, 123
compounds, 26, 28, 70, 73
comprehension, 159
compression, 79, 131, 132, 135, 136, 138, 142, 152
conception, 125
conditioning, 32, 119
condyloma, 103
congestive heart failure, 70
conjunctivitis, 15
connective tissue, 25, 157, 170
consciousness, 80
consensus, x, 11, 84, 85, 132, 133, 135, 149, 154, 159
constellation of mechanism-based, vii, 9
constituents, 120
contact dermatitis, 83
contour, 126
contracture, 140
controlled studies, 5, 97
controlled trials, vii, 9, 11
controversial, 52, 83, 142, 155, 158
controversies, 150, 153, 161
cooling, 29, 34, 155, 156, 157
coordination, 23
copper, 57
corneal ulcer, 15
correlation, 42, 44, 91
correlations, 113
cortex, 22
corticosteroid cream, 13
corticosteroid paste, vii, 9
corticosteroid therapy, 190
corticosteroids, 5, 7, 11, 12, 15, 17, 27, 55, 155
cosmetic, ix, 28, 58, 117, 118, 119, 120, 121, 122, 123, 124, 125, 126, 184
cosmetics, 127
cost, 79
cotton, 57
covering, 22, 86, 91, 184, 186, 187, 188, 190, 191, 192, 193, 194
CPT, 76

cranium, 52
criticism, 157
crowns, 125
cryosurgery, 142
cryotherapy, 11, 145, 148
CSF, 156, 161
culture, 13, 25, 86
cure, viii, 24, 51, 110, 180
cures, 14, 25, 36, 58
Cutaneous metastases, ix, 95, 96, 97, 98, 103, 104,
    106, 107, 108, 109, 110, 111, 112, 114
cuticle, 22
cyanotic, 177
cycles, 3, 38, 40, 42, 43, 45, 67
cyclical process, 23
cycling, 30
cyclooxygenase, 5, 49
cyclophosphamide, 25, 28, 34, 40, 64, 73
cyclosporine, 29
cytokines, 27
cytosine, 31, 34, 74
cytoskeleton, 22
cytostatic-induced alopecia, viii, 21, 26, 29
cytotoxic agents, 42, 55, 162
cytotoxicity, 3, 13

D

daily living, 36, 136, 185
damages, viii, 79
dandruff, 126
data collection, 159
debridement, 158, 159
defects, 126
deficiencies, 53, 85
deficiency, 60, 61, 68, 74, 176
degradation, 155
deltoid, 140
dementia, 176
demographic characteristics, 86
Department of Health and Human Services, 185
dependent variable, 91
deposition, ix, 100, 139, 140, 192
deposits, 131, 173, 174, 176
depth, 38, 145
derivatives, 71, 176
dermabrasion, 126
dermal injury, ix, 139
dermatitis, 19, 41, 56, 60, 61, 62, 68, 69, 70, 71, 75,
    83, 101, 153, 165, 167, 171, 172, 176, 186, 189
dermatologic treatment, vii, 9
dermatologist, 11, 36, 183
dermatology, 23, 87, 126

dermatomyositis, x, 163, 170, 179, 180
dermatosis, 24, 31, 180
dermis, 4, 22, 81, 121, 140, 145, 183, 192, 193
desensitization, 73
destruction, 14, 24, 40, 81, 152, 157, 192
detachment, 97, 193
detection, ix, 4, 95, 96, 97, 113
detoxification, 58
developed countries, 132
diabetes, 152, 175
diarrhea, 68, 71, 72, 158, 175, 176
diet, 57
differential diagnosis, 109
diffusion, 121
dilation, 4
dimerization, 72
dimethylsulfoxide, 156, 157, 162
discharges, 106
disclosure, 28
discomfort, 3, 4, 46, 81, 154, 155, 189, 192
diseases, 74, 163, 165, 167, 176, 178, 179, 181
dislocation, 152, 153
disorder, 109, 170, 186, 187, 188, 189, 190, 191,
    192, 193, 194
dispersion, 157
disposition, 162
distribution, 47, 96, 98, 110, 178, 187
DNA, 25, 53, 55, 63, 64, 67, 69, 70, 71, 150, 151,
    155, 157
DNA repair, 55
docetaxel, 2, 7, 25, 42, 43, 45, 48, 49, 55, 61, 70, 75,
    150, 153, 155
dogs, 7
dosage, 25, 46, 68, 123
dosing, 64, 93
double-blind trial, 18
drainage, 80, 85, 86, 125, 133, 135, 136, 138
dressings, 55, 56, 83, 125, 142
drug withdrawal, 4
drug-induced lupus, 12
drugs, vii, viii, x, 1, 10, 25, 26, 28, 35, 36, 38, 40, 42,
    43, 44, 55, 56, 63, 64, 67, 69, 70, 149, 150, 151,
    152, 154, 155, 156, 157, 158, 159, 161, 162, 171,
    178
drying, 11, 14, 137
dyspnea, 72

E

eczema, vii, 9, 10, 13, 14, 15, 16, 54, 98, 164
edema, vi, ix, 2, 129, 131, 132, 133, 135, 136, 138,
    152, 174, 176, 189, 190, 193
education, 4, 11, 135

EGFR-targeted therapies, vii, 9
elaboration, 133
elbows, 3
electrolyte, 67, 186, 187, 188
electron, 7, 38, 48, 60
electron microscopy, 7
elongation, 23
emulsifying agents, 117
emulsions, 117, 119
encoding, 92
endometriosis, 103
energy, 85, 145
enlargement, 110, 129
environment, 80, 83
environmental factors, ix, 139, 140
enzyme, 68, 70, 122, 157
enzymes, 68, 71
eosinophilia, 68, 74, 168
epidemiology, 80
epidermal growth factor receptor (EGFR), viii, 10, 19, 32, 35, 36, 49, 92
epidermis, 10, 22, 26, 81, 89, 120, 121, 192
epithelial cells, 90
epithelium, 22, 37, 40
equipment, 152
erlonitib.-immunochemistry, ix
erysipelas, 3, 100, 103, 131
erythema gyratum repens, x, 163, 179
erythema multiforme, 71
erythema nodosum, 104, 113, 167
erythrocytes, 100
esophageal cancer, 107, 180
esophagus, 96, 110, 167
estrogen, 27, 179
etiology, ix, 129, 136, 145, 167, 170
Europe, 11, 18, 59, 62, 86, 158
evidence, vii, 2, 9, 10, 11, 16, 29, 57, 59, 80, 83, 85, 159, 161, 164, 171
evolution, x, 28, 52, 132, 155, 163, 180
excision, 14, 110, 136, 142, 145, 162
excretion, 176
exercise, 136, 138
exposure, viii, 4, 11, 42, 51, 52, 53, 55, 57, 58, 59, 91, 152, 153, 177
extensor, 170
extracellular matrix, 22, 30
extraction, 14
extracts, 57
extravasation, x, 75, 97, 149, 150, 152, 153, 154, 155, 156, 157, 158, 159, 160, 161, 162
exudate, 83, 85, 167

F

facies, 175
families, 153
family history, 145
fascia, 81, 193
fat, 131, 143, 158, 177, 192
FDA, 74, 158, 162
fever, 68, 69
fiber, 34
fibroblast growth factor, 28
fibroblasts, 25, 122
fibrosarcoma, 107
fibrosis, 69, 122, 133, 155
filters, 58
filtration, 130
fistulas, 86
fluid, 117, 129, 130, 131, 133, 186, 187, 189
fluorescence, 158, 162
foams, 119
folate, 67
folic acid, 67
follicle, 10, 22, 23, 25, 30, 31, 90
folliculitis, 10, 13, 44, 90
food, 57, 81, 93
food intake, 81
formation, viii, 30, 35, 40, 80, 92, 132, 145, 147, 152
fractures, 59
fragility, 41, 72
fragments, 41
France, 1, 51, 79, 126
free radicals, 57, 157
friction, 4, 14, 79, 80, 83, 84
fungal infection, 137, 142
fungus, 90

G

gallbladder, 165, 171
gastrin, 107
gastrointestinal tract, 100, 102, 180
gel, 11, 84
gender differences, 2
genes, 92
genetic predisposition, 52
genitourinary tract, 98, 101
Germany, 95
gingival, 104
gland, 4, 74, 101, 109, 164
glaucoma, 189
glioblastoma, 93
glioblastoma multiforme, 93

glucagon, 173, 175
glue, 14
glycosaminoglycans, 22
grades, 82
grading, 3, 13, 26, 36, 47, 86, 89, 91, 185
granulomas, 42, 43, 46, 110
growth, viii, 10, 18, 19, 21, 23, 24, 26, 27, 28, 29,
    30, 32, 33, 34, 35, 36, 37, 40, 42, 45, 48, 49, 64,
    76, 83, 86, 87, 89, 90, 92, 93, 132, 140, 156, 167,
    170, 171, 178, 186, 187
growth factor, viii, 10, 18, 19, 26, 28, 32, 33, 35, 36,
    42, 48, 49, 76, 89, 92, 93, 156, 167
growth rate, 23
guidance, 31, 85, 158
guidelines, vii, 9, 16, 19, 83, 84, 154, 155, 157, 159,
    160
gynecomastia, x, 163, 179, 180

H

hair, vii, 9, 10, 17, 19, 21, 22, 23, 24, 25, 26, 27, 28,
    29, 30, 31, 32, 33, 34, 44, 49, 64, 72, 73, 90, 92,
    106, 119, 120, 121, 122, 126, 170, 171, 178, 186,
    187, 188
hair cells, 29
hair effluvium, viii, 21
hair fibres, vii, 21
hair follicle, 10, 22, 23, 24, 25, 28, 29, 30, 31, 34, 64,
    92, 106
hair loss, 21, 23, 24, 31, 34, 122, 126, 186
hair matrix, viii, 21, 22, 25
half-life, 29
hand-foot syndrome (HFS), vii, 1, 68
hardness, 81, 192
harmful effects, 58
hazards, 31
HCC, 108
head and neck cancer, 10, 12
headache, 29
healing, 3, 55, 83, 85, 87, 133, 139, 140, 146, 157,
    158
health, viii, 34, 79, 80
heart disease, 181
height, 85
hemochromatosis, 175
hemorrhage, 49, 71, 190
hepatitis, 12, 33
hepatocellular carcinoma, 110, 114, 180
herpes, 13, 14, 109, 126
herpes simplex, 13, 14
herpes zoster, 109
hidradenitis suppurativa, 109
hirsutism, x, 21, 29, 163, 171, 178, 180

histology, 101, 106, 141
history, 67, 80
hormones, viii, 51
hospitalization, vii, ix, 1, 2, 129, 135, 185, 194
host, 85
human, 25, 29, 30, 31, 34, 93, 120, 123, 124, 125,
    133
human body, 120, 125
human health, 120
humidity, 83
hydatidiform mole, 32
hydrocortisone, 156, 157
hygiene, 17, 119, 124
hyperandrogenism, 173
hyperpigmentation, vii, 9, 10, 11, 12, 14, 17, 64, 69,
    70, 71, 131, 145, 152, 164, 192
hypersensitivity, 64, 67, 71, 73, 152, 154, 167, 172,
    193
hypertension, 72
hypertrichosis, viii, x, 21, 22, 28, 29, 33, 163, 171,
    178, 179, 180
hypertrichosis lanuginose, 33
hypertrophic osteoarhtropathy, x, 163
hypertrophic scars, ix, 110, 139, 140, 142, 145, 148
hypertrophy, 188
hypodermis, 22, 121
hypokalemia, 174
hypotension, 72, 80
hypothermia, viii, 21, 29
hypothesis, 3, 53, 69
hysterectomy, 137

I

iatrogenic, x, 110, 149
ideal, 83, 84, 118, 155
identification, 152, 158
idiopathic, 167, 170
image, 30, 100
immune response, 130
immune system, viii, 51, 130
immunomodulator, 29
immunosuppression, 34
immunosuppressive drugs, 170
immunotherapy, 93
implants, 125
in vitro, 31, 57, 62, 157
in vivo, 25, 62
incidence, ix, 2, 5, 12, 42, 43, 46, 47, 52, 53, 68, 70,
    80, 86, 90, 95, 98, 132, 133, 140, 142, 149, 160
Indians, 145
indirect measure, 91
individuals, ix, 52, 53, 139, 140

inducer, 29
induction, 3, 7, 12
induration, 81, 100, 152, 192
industry, 121, 124
infection, x, 14, 44, 46, 79, 85, 133, 139, 140, 147, 163, 167
inflammation, 11, 13, 44, 69, 74, 100, 140, 152, 153, 155, 186
inflammatory bowel disease, 168
inflammatory cells, 155
inflammatory disease, 167
infundibulum, 22
ingestion, 57
ingredients, 120, 124
inguinal, 102, 107, 108, 132, 134, 135, 137, 138
inhibition, 3, 5, 10, 19, 23, 34, 43, 48, 76, 89, 90, 92
inhibitor, vii, 5, 6, 9, 10, 11, 12, 13, 14, 16, 17, 18, 19, 29, 32, 44, 45, 46, 47, 48, 49, 68, 69, 71, 76, 77, 90, 92, 93, 157, 162
initiation, ix, 12, 24, 29, 44, 95, 96
injections, 125, 142, 145
injuries, 150, 156, 158, 159, 160, 162
injury, viii, ix, 35, 36, 40, 85, 125, 139, 140, 146, 150, 153, 155, 158, 161, 162
institutions, x, 149
insulin, 165, 188
insulin resistance, 165
integration, 184
interface, viii, 79, 80, 84
interferon, 28, 33, 61, 142, 145
internist, 11
intervention, 24, 85, 158, 183, 185, 186, 188, 189, 190, 194
intestine, 96
intramuscular injection, 161
intraocular, 189
intraocular pressure, 189
intravenously, 158, 159
involution, 23
iodine, 14
ionizing radiations, viii, 21, 142
ipsilateral, 153
iridium, 145
iron, x, 58, 183
iron oxide, x, 183
irradiation, 24, 60, 69, 147
ischemic tissue damages, viii, 79
isolation, 36
issues, 152
Italy, 41

J

joints, 170

K

kaposi sarcoma, 60, 61
keloid, 140, 141
keloids, ix, 139, 140, 142, 145, 147, 148
keratin, 37
keratinocytes, 3, 4, 22, 25, 38, 51, 90
keratosis, 166
kidney, 52, 96, 97, 100, 106, 110, 165, 171
kinase activity, 44, 72

L

lack of control, 154
large intestine, 96
laryngeal cancer, 110
larynx, 52, 97, 114
lasers, 183
latency, 23
laws, 121
lead, vii, x, 3, 23, 25, 36, 42, 43, 54, 55, 67, 68, 80, 108, 142, 149, 153, 155, 159, 163, 179
leakage, 149
legislation, 119, 124, 125, 127
legs, 103, 166, 176
lesions, ix, 3, 10, 12, 13, 48, 91, 95, 97, 98, 100, 101, 103, 104, 105, 106, 107, 108, 109, 110, 113, 114, 126, 140, 142, 158, 162, 167, 168, 170, 175, 176, 184, 187, 190, 194
leukemia, 60, 74, 96, 104, 109, 113, 171
lice, 124
lichen, 100
ligand, 27, 44, 72
light, 7, 53, 54, 57, 117, 168, 173, 176, 184, 190
lipodystrophy, 165
lipolysis, 122
liposuction, 136, 138
liquids, 119
liver, 64, 68, 71, 96, 108, 110, 158, 172, 173, 176
liver cancer, 110
liver disease, 172
liver enzymes, 158
liver metastases, 176
localization, 4, 110, 155
longitudinal melanonychia, viii, 35, 38, 40
lower limb edema, ix, 129, 135
lung cancer, 10, 15, 33, 42, 48, 67, 68, 69, 71, 74, 76, 92, 93, 97, 106, 110, 165, 173, 174, 181

lung function, 69
lupus, 100, 173
lycopene, 57
lymph, 104, 106, 130, 131, 132, 133, 135, 136, 137, 138, 153, 167
lymph node, 104, 106, 130, 132, 133, 136, 137, 138, 153, 167
lymphangioma, 100, 109
lymphangitis, 131
lymphatic system, ix, 129, 130, 131, 132
lymphedema, 131, 132, 133, 136, 137, 152
lymphocytes, 10
lymphoma, 52, 67, 69, 76, 96, 104, 113, 181
lysis, 66

M

macroglossia, 176
magnesium, 58
magnetic resonance, 159, 162
magnetic resonance imaging, (MRI), 159, 162
majority, x, 15, 16, 26, 63, 97, 100, 102, 106, 107, 117, 119, 123, 149, 159
malaise, 167
malignancy, x, 76, 97, 98, 101, 106, 109, 110, 141, 163, 164, 165, 167, 171, 173, 179, 180, 181
malignant cells, 100
malignant melanoma, 33, 59, 96, 97, 112, 181
malignant tumors, 93
malnutrition, 80, 85
man, 25, 57, 140
management, vii, viii, ix, x, 1, 2, 3, 11, 12, 18, 19, 22, 31, 33, 37, 47, 48, 49, 60, 63, 75, 85, 86, 89, 132, 133, 138, 149, 150, 154, 155, 157, 158, 159, 161, 162, 167, 171
manganese, 57
mapping, 138
marketing, 119
masking, 126
mass, 134, 141
mastectomy, 145
mastitis, 142, 147
materials, 125
matrix, viii, ix, 14, 21, 22, 23, 25, 36, 37, 38, 40, 43, 45, 139, 140
matter, vii, 23, 57, 107, 155
measurements, 53, 62, 85
median, 42, 45, 55, 137, 153
mediastinitis, 152
medical, ix, x, 10, 86, 117, 118, 122, 123, 124, 125, 126, 127, 149, 159, 183, 184, 186, 188
medicine, 72
medulla, 22, 30

melanin, 38, 45, 52, 173, 174, 192
melanocytes, viii, 21, 22, 25, 27, 38, 45, 47
melanoma, ix, 45, 52, 53, 57, 59, 95, 96, 97, 100, 102, 104, 106, 110, 126, 132, 133, 137, 138, 173
menadione, 12, 19
mental health, 132
mental state, 80
mesothelioma, 68
meta-analysis, 59, 85, 87
metabolism, 67
metabolites, 64, 67, 68, 73, 155
metabolized, 68, 150
metastasis, ix, 24, 95, 97, 98, 100, 101, 102, 105, 106, 107, 108, 109, 110, 111, 112, 113, 114, 115, 132
metastatic cancer, 111
metastatic disease, 97, 102, 108, 109, 111, 175
mice, 10, 31, 34, 92, 162
microcirculation, 80
microorganisms, 85
microscopy, 158, 162
mimicry, ix, 95, 109
minoxidil, viii, 21
misconceptions, ix, 117
mitosis, 4, 43
mitoxantrone, 40, 64, 151, 160
MLD, 135, 136
models, 25, 29, 98, 154
modifications, vii, 21, 27, 38, 44
moisture, 80, 81, 83
molecules, 32, 36, 71, 121, 122
monoclonal antibody, 33, 72, 92, 93
morbidity, viii, 43, 63, 137, 138
morphea, 100, 109
morphology, 107, 108
mortality, viii, 52, 53, 59, 79
mortality rate, viii, 52, 79
mucosa, 10, 64, 102
mucosal changes, vii, 9, 17
mucous membrane, 120, 190, 193
multiple myeloma, 32, 71, 165, 170, 176, 178
multiples, 44
multipotent, 25, 31
muscles, 170
myalgia, 72

N

nail biting, 46
nail polish, 45
narcotics, 188, 190
National Institutes of Health, vi, 185
nausea, 67, 68, 69, 70, 71, 72, 158

necrosis, 4, 74, 75, 80, 81, 150, 152, 154, 158, 161, 162, 167, 168, 174, 175, 176, 177, 192
neoplasm, 24, 28, 98, 106, 110, 111, 132, 164
nerve, 5, 7, 152
nerve fibers, 5, 7
neuroblastoma, 104, 105
neurotoxicity, 67, 70
neutropenia, 45, 68, 158
nevus, 62, 103, 113, 115
New Zealand, 53
niacin, 176
nitrogen, 157
nodes, 104, 132, 133
nodules, ix, 70, 95, 98, 99, 100, 101, 102, 103, 104, 105, 106, 107, 108, 110, 113, 114, 141, 142, 164, 173, 176, 177
Norton Scale, viii, 79, 80
Norway, 53
NSAIDs, 188, 190
nuclei, 40
nucleic acid, 66, 150
nuisance, 48
nurses, 80, 152, 153, 154, 159, 160
nursing care, 160
nutrition, 80, 85, 87
nutritional status, x, 85, 139

O

obesity, 131, 152
obstruction, ix, 129, 131, 132
occlusion, 14, 17, 153
oedema, 13, 41, 55, 72, 73, 85, 136
oesophageal, 67, 89
oil, 11, 12, 13, 17
old age, 80
omega-3, 57
oncogenesis, 26
onycholysis, viii, 35, 36, 40, 43, 46, 48, 49, 54, 69, 71, 75
onychomadesis, viii, 35, 45
operations, 126
optic neuritis, 190
oral antibiotic, 191
oral cavity, 96, 103, 106, 120
oral cefuroxim axetil, vii, 9
oral minocycline, vii, 9, 12, 15, 16, 18
organ, 34, 98
organism, 86, 124
organs, 100, 106, 109, 120, 130, 176
osteoarthropathy, 179
osteogenic sarcoma, 61, 107
osteomyelitis, 86

ototoxicity, 67
outpatients, 153
ovarian cancer, 67, 69, 71, 110
overlap, 118, 150
overproduction, 175
oxidation, 25

P

Pacific, 70
paclitaxel, 7, 25, 28, 31, 42, 43, 48, 49, 54, 55, 60, 61, 70, 71, 150, 153, 155, 157, 160
paediatric patients, 40
pain, 2, 10, 14, 36, 46, 68, 79, 85, 140, 142, 145, 150, 152, 153, 154, 155, 158, 189, 190, 192
palliative, 7, 24
palmoplantar erythrodysesthesia, vii, 1
pancreas, 96, 100, 106, 114, 171
pancreatic cancer, 69, 107
pancreatitis, 176
paracentesis, 103
parallel, 38, 40, 91, 145, 165, 170, 173, 179, 192
Paraneoplastic skin manifestations, x, 163, 173, 180
paraneoplastic syndrome, 164, 170, 172, 179, 180
paresthesias, 2
paronychia, vii, 9, 10, 13, 14, 17, 19, 27, 32, 41, 43, 44, 45, 48, 49, 71
parotid, 100, 110, 114
pathogenesis, viii, ix, 31, 35, 38, 43, 44, 48, 139, 140, 150, 160, 165, 167
pathology, 76, 111
pathophysiological, x, 163, 173, 180
pathophysiology, 18, 49, 72, 164, 166
pathways, 31, 133, 134, 135, 138
patient care, 159
pellagra, 54, 173, 176
pelvis, 84, 107, 114
pemphigus, 68, 74, 180
penicillin, 13
penis, 108, 114
peptide, 29
perfusion, viii, 21, 25, 29, 56
pericardiocentesis, 115
peripheral neuropathy, 71, 152
permeability, 157
permit, 117, 153
pernio, 104
PET, 125
pharmaceuticals, 127
pharmacokinetics, 91, 93
phenotype, 90, 91
Philadelphia, 76, 137
phlebitis, 150, 152, 154

photosensitivity, 12, 53, 59, 60, 190
photosynthesis, 53
physical activity, 81
physical therapy, 137
physicians, 67
physiology, ix, 129, 130
physiopathology, vii, ix, 1, 40, 129, 136
pigmentation, x, 45, 47, 56, 69, 73, 100, 145, 163, 164, 166, 173, 174, 180
pilot study, 34, 86, 147
pityriasis rosea, 72
placebo, 18, 76, 161
plants, 70
plaque, 26, 70, 75, 100, 141
platinum, 66, 67, 150
pneumonitis, 61
polycythemia, 171
polycythemia vera, 171
polymorphism, 22
polymorphisms, 91
polyps, 181
population, 2, 22, 126, 137, 158, 159
population control, 137
population group, 2
porphyria, 72
porphyrins, 60
portal venous system, 98
Portugal, 39
prediction tools, viii, 79, 80
pregnancy, 123, 167
prejudice, 28
preparation, 12, 58, 120
preservation, x, 149
pressure sore, 84
pressure ulcers, viii, 79, 86, 87
prevention, vii, ix, 1, 4, 24, 29, 57, 62, 79, 83, 84, 85, 86, 87, 125, 126, 153, 157, 159, 161, 162
primary tumor, ix, 95, 97, 103, 106, 110, 132
principles, 11
professionals, 146, 150, 154
progenitor cells, 7
prognosis, 3, 47, 110, 171
proliferation, 3, 22, 43, 69, 90, 97, 140
prophylactic, vii, 9, 12, 18
prophylaxis, 5
prostate cancer, 106, 108
prostate carcinoma, 106, 114
protection, 14, 16, 17, 57, 58, 62, 121, 153, 159
protective role, 53
proteins, 26, 66, 130, 131
proteinuria, 72
proteolytic enzyme, 157
prototype, 70

pruritus, 67, 91, 142, 165, 168, 172, 179, 186, 187, 191
psoriasis, 36, 38
psychological distress, 22
psychological functions, 123
puberty, 178
public health, 53
purpura, 104, 176, 177, 193
pus, 86
putative cause, 173
pyoderma gangrenosum, 168
pyogenic, viii, 13, 14, 16, 35, 41, 44, 48, 109, 114
pyogenic granuloma, viii, 13, 14, 16, 35, 41, 44, 48, 109, 114
pyrimidine, 67, 68

Q

quality of life, vii, viii, x, 1, 2, 9, 10, 17, 34, 35, 36, 42, 47, 64, 68, 132, 136, 138, 149, 184

R

race, 2, 140, 188
radiation, 19, 31, 36, 53, 55, 56, 59, 60, 61, 62, 67, 68, 69, 70, 71, 73, 75, 93, 131, 133, 142, 147, 152, 153
radiation damage, 152
radiation therapy, 31, 55, 61, 75, 93, 131, 133, 142
radical formation, 150
radio, 31
radiotherapy, 12, 19, 24, 52, 55, 58, 68, 133, 135, 137, 142, 145, 147
rash, ix, 10, 12, 13, 18, 19, 27, 53, 64, 67, 68, 69, 71, 72, 73, 76, 89, 90, 91, 92, 93, 169, 170, 191
reactions, vii, viii, 9, 11, 12, 13, 18, 27, 31, 33, 47, 54, 55, 61, 63, 64, 65, 67, 68, 70, 71, 72, 73, 75, 76, 90, 110, 152, 153, 154, 159, 160
reactive oxygen, 57
reactivity, 73
reading, 120
reality, 118
reasoning, 121
recall, 31, 55, 56, 60, 61, 62, 65, 67, 68, 69, 70, 71, 73, 74, 75, 153, 161
reception, 89
receptors, 10, 27, 29, 42, 48, 72, 91
recognition, vii, viii, 1, 2, 63, 85, 154, 159, 179, 180
recommendations, 11, 17, 45, 154, 157, 160, 161
recovery, 79, 157
rectum, 52, 53, 67, 100, 102, 106
recurrence, 46, 85, 141, 142, 145, 146, 148

regenerate, 5, 22, 133
regeneration, 23
regression, 22, 23, 25
regrowth, 25
rehabilitation, 80, 135
relevance, 87
relief, 14, 84, 173, 176
renal cell carcinoma, 3, 73, 76, 92, 103, 106, 114
repair, ix, x, 24, 42, 139, 140, 183
replication, 71
researchers, 145
resection, 153, 175
resistance, 13, 25, 31, 83, 138, 154
resolution, 90, 140, 142
response, 5, 12, 17, 28, 31, 36, 44, 55, 61, 71, 76, 91, 93, 111, 147, 164, 167
restoration, 161
restrictions, 120, 124
rheumatoid arthritis, 168
rings, 168
risk, viii, x, 28, 32, 42, 43, 52, 53, 57, 59, 69, 79, 80, 81, 84, 85, 86, 108, 133, 137, 138, 139, 140, 142, 147, 152, 154, 159, 160
risk assessment, 80, 86
risk factors, x, 80, 138, 139, 140, 152
risks, 12, 53, 85, 142, 147
rituximab, 72
RNA, 69, 70
rods, 86
root, 27
rosacea, 12, 19, 124, 126
routes, 107
RPR, 113
rules, x, 119, 149, 152

S

sacrum, 80
safety, 70, 74, 119
salivary gland, 53, 96, 107
salts, 119
saturation, 91
scaling, 100, 166, 171, 172
scanning electron microscopy, 49
scientific understanding, 159
scleroderma, 71, 103
sclerosis, 170, 176
scrotum, 102
sebaceous cyst, 114
seborrheic dermatitis, 126
secretion, 167, 173, 174, 175, 176, 178, 179
seeding, 113, 115
selenium, 57, 58

self-confidence, 126
self-esteem, 10
sensation, 135, 152, 157, 189, 190, 192
sensitivity, 13, 55, 60, 65, 68, 80, 190
sensors, 84
sepsis, 43
serotonin, 173
serum, 29, 53, 85
serum albumin, 85
services, 125, 126
sex, 97
sexual behaviour, 178
shape, viii, 21, 22, 26, 29
shear, 79, 80, 81, 84
sheep, 73
showing, 22, 99, 103, 145, 159
side effects, vii, viii, 9, 10, 12, 13, 32, 33, 35, 36, 38, 42, 44, 46, 47, 48, 59, 60, 61, 63, 69, 70, 71, 72, 73, 76, 89, 92, 145, 157, 158, 183
signaling pathway, 3
signalling, 91
signs, x, 14, 18, 49, 67, 100, 111, 152, 154, 163, 164, 174, 179, 180, 192, 193
silk, 57
silver, 18, 45, 46, 175
simulation, 114
skin cancer, viii, 51, 52, 53, 57, 58, 59, 109, 126, 138, 165, 168
skin grafting, 85
skin toxicity, vii, 1, 2, 9, 10, 11, 12, 13, 16, 17, 18, 33, 36, 47, 49, 61, 72, 155, 161, 162
Social Security, 28
society, 153
sodium, 156, 157, 161
soft tissue tumors, 103
software, 125
solid tumors, 3, 89, 92, 93, 96, 167, 170, 171
solution, 14, 45, 117, 157
species, 57
specifications, 119
spindle, 141
squamous cell, 19, 32, 52, 57, 59, 67, 76, 96, 101, 103, 106, 107, 108, 110, 112, 114, 133, 142, 152, 165, 167, 173
squamous cell carcinoma, 19, 32, 52, 57, 59, 67, 76, 96, 101, 103, 106, 107, 108, 110, 112, 114, 133, 142, 165, 167, 173
stability, 58
stabilization, 140
Staphylococcus aureus, vii, 9, 13, 17, 86
stasis, 97
state, 130, 131
states, 120, 121, 131

steel, 152
stem cells, 22, 30, 55
sterile, 10, 13, 125, 156
steroid cream, 14
steroids, vii, 9, 13, 15, 137, 167, 168
Stevens-Johnson syndrome, 193
stomach, 52, 53, 67, 96, 100, 106, 109, 110, 165, 181
stomatitis, 15, 68, 70, 73, 158
storage, 53
stress, 24, 153
striae, 192
stroke, 105, 188
stroma, 100, 157
structure, vii, 21, 22, 67, 71, 192
style, 186
subacute, 45
subcutaneous injection, 188
subcutaneous tissue, 81, 131, 145, 157, 186, 187, 188, 189, 190, 191, 192, 193, 194
substrate, 157
success rate, 157
sulphur, 92
Sun, 14, 16, 30, 51, 52, 53, 55, 56, 57, 58
superior vena cava, 152
superior vena cava syndrome, 152
supplementation, 53, 59, 62, 85
suppression, 67, 68, 69, 158
surface area, 187
surgical intervention, 24, 158
surgical removal, 24, 158
surgical resection, 158
surgical technique, 132
surrogates, x, 163, 180
surveillance, 67
survival, 91, 97, 110, 137
survivors, 147
susceptibility, 25
suture, 145
sweat, 74, 122
swelling, 2, 53, 68, 101, 110, 131, 135, 152, 153, 154, 189
symptoms, vii, x, 3, 4, 5, 9, 14, 15, 17, 68, 91, 150, 152, 154, 163, 179, 180, 185, 187, 191, 192, 193, 194
syndrome, vii, viii, x, 1, 3, 4, 6, 7, 27, 31, 32, 60, 61, 63, 65, 68, 69, 70, 71, 72, 73, 74, 75, 137, 163, 164, 165, 166, 167, 168, 171, 172, 173, 175, 176, 177, 179, 180, 181, 189, 193
synergistic effect, 43, 131
synthesis, viii, 23, 51, 63, 64, 69, 70, 122, 176
systemic lupus erythematosus, 73
systolic blood pressure, 29

T

T cell, 165, 171
tamoxifen, 28, 61, 179
target, 2, 24, 42, 71, 157, 187
taxane, 25, 40, 43
techniques, x, 12, 85, 149, 155, 183, 184
technology, 29
teeth, 64, 119, 120
telangiectasia, vii, 9, 10, 12, 17, 184
temperature, 4, 98, 111, 188
tendons, 152
testicular cancer, 67, 69, 160
testing, 73, 154
tetracyclines, 12, 13, 14
texture, 22, 26, 117, 186
TGF, 90, 142
therapeutic use, 76
therapist, 136
therapy, vii, ix, x, 1, 2, 4, 6, 7, 9, 11, 12, 13, 14, 18, 25, 27, 31, 33, 38, 44, 48, 49, 60, 61, 67, 71, 73, 74, 75, 76, 95, 96, 136, 139, 142, 143, 144, 145, 157, 163, 164, 166, 167, 168, 171, 179, 190
thinning, 24, 38, 44, 192
thoracostomy, 101
thorax, 70
thrombocytopenia, 40
thrombosis, 152
thyroid, 96, 108, 110, 164, 176
thyroid cancer, 164
tin, 2, 68, 189
tinea capitis, 27
tissue, viii, 24, 41, 46, 68, 79, 80, 81, 83, 85, 97, 101, 110, 131, 136, 140, 150, 152, 153, 154, 157, 158, 159, 161, 162, 183, 192
tissue plasminogen activator, 153, 161
titanium, 58
TNF, 168
tonsils, 100
topical antibiotics, 15, 83, 156
topical metronidazole, vii, 9, 11, 12, 15, 17
topical steroids, vii, 9, 15, 137
tourniquet, viii, 21, 29
toxic effect, viii, 63
toxicity, vii, viii, 1, 2, 9, 10, 11, 12, 13, 16, 17, 18, 19, 25, 33, 36, 38, 42, 43, 44, 46, 47, 48, 49, 61, 63, 64, 65, 67, 68, 69, 70, 71, 72, 73, 75, 155, 161, 162, 163
toxoplasmosis, 167
trace elements, 57, 85
trachea, 110
transcription, 69
transduction, 26

transitional cell carcinoma, 107, 114
transmission, 119
transplantation, 32
transport, 130, 131
trastuzumab therapy, 60
trauma, 44, 46, 111, 131, 140, 145, 190
treatment, vii, viii, ix, x, 1, 3, 4, 5, 7, 9, 10, 11, 12,
    13, 14, 16, 17, 19, 21, 24, 25, 26, 27, 28, 29, 30,
    32, 33, 35, 36, 38, 42, 43, 44, 45, 46, 48, 49, 51,
    55, 56, 58, 63, 64, 66, 67, 68, 69, 70, 71, 72, 73,
    74, 76, 79, 83, 84, 85, 87, 89, 90, 91, 92, 124,
    125, 126, 129, 131, 132, 133, 135, 136, 137, 138,
    139, 142, 143, 145, 146, 147, 148, 149, 152, 153,
    154, 155, 156, 157, 158, 159, 160, 161, 162, 170,
    176, 184
trial, 3, 18, 32, 34, 59, 62, 74, 75, 76, 90, 92, 93, 161
trichocytes, viii, 21, 22
trichomegaly, viii, 10, 21, 28, 33
trochanter, 84
tryptophan, 176
tumor, ix, x, 3, 6, 10, 13, 26, 30, 34, 68, 69, 89, 91,
    92, 93, 95, 96, 97, 99, 100, 101, 103, 105, 106,
    108, 109, 110, 133, 141, 163, 164, 165, 167, 170,
    171, 173, 174, 175, 178, 179, 180
tumor cells, ix, 68, 95, 96, 100, 103, 105, 107, 110
tumor development, 3
tumor growth, 26, 34
tumors, 28, 69, 72, 92, 97, 100, 104, 107, 108, 109,
    110, 111, 113, 114, 115, 132, 141, 165, 170, 173,
    174, 175, 176, 178, 179
tyrosine, vii, viii, 9, 10, 26, 28, 32, 44, 63, 72, 73, 76,
    77, 92, 93
tyrosine kinase inhibitors, vii, viii, 9, 10, 28, 63, 72,
    73

U

ulcer, viii, 79, 80, 81, 83, 84, 85, 86, 87, 167, 192
united, 11
United States, 11
urea, 66
urethra, 107, 114
urinary bladder, 96
urinary tract, 107, 114
urine, 81, 157, 174
urticaria, 64, 71, 181
USA, 36, 52, 92
uterus, 100, 165, 168
UV light, 158
UV radiation, 55

V

vagina, 15
validation, 87
variables, 145
variations, 11, 149
vascular system, 130
vascularization, 55
vasculature, 3
vasculitis, x, 69, 74, 76, 100, 163, 177, 180, 181
vasoconstriction, 29, 105, 155
vein, 133, 152, 153, 154, 158
vessels, 36, 42, 100, 132, 152, 193
vitamin B6, 5
vitamin C, 85
vitamin D, viii, 29, 51, 53, 59
vitamin E, 5, 7
vitamin K, 12, 19
vitamins, 7, 57, 58, 85
vitiligo, 124, 126
vomiting, 67, 68, 69, 70, 71, 158
vulva, 103, 108, 109

W

walking, 2, 4, 14
water, 11, 13, 17, 45, 84, 147, 156
weakness, 132, 170
wear, 38, 57, 136
weeping, 53
weight loss, 85
withdrawal, 3, 90
World Health Organization (WHO), 2, 3, 25, 26
wound dehiscence, 146
wound healing, x, 72, 83, 86, 87, 89, 139, 147, 156,
    161
wound infection, 85, 87, 133, 140, 146

X

xerosis, vii, 9, 11, 13, 16, 17, 44, 72, 126, 170, 179

Y

yeast, 14

Z

zinc, 57, 58, 85
zinc oxide, 58